How to be Stylish and Chic

A Quick Guidebook on Dressing Stylish and Being Chic

Lisa Lewis

PUBLISHED BY:
Lisa Lewis

TABLE OF CONTENTS

CHAPTER 1: HOW TO BE STYLISH AND CHIC 6

Introduction 6

CHAPTER 2: GENERAL CLOTHING STYLES 8

How to Create the Stylish Look 9

Becoming More Stylish 11

How Do You Dress Up in a Chic and Stylish Way? 13

How Do You Choose Trendy Fashionable Clothes Ideally Suited for You?....15

What are the Key Pieces in a Chic and Stylish Wardrobe? 16

CHAPTER 3: STYLISH DRESSING 21

Tips on How to Dress Like a Stylish Teen 22

How Can You Look Really Stylish and Chic at Prom? 23

How to Dress Stylish in College 24

What to Wear on a Company Dinner? 25

How to Dress Stylishly in Plus-Sized Clothing 27

Layering Clothes in a Stylish Way 29

How to Find Trendy and Stylish Maternity Clothes 31

Who Says New Moms can't be Stylish and Chic? 34

How to Build an Outfit around a Chic Accessory 37

CHAPTER 4: THE STYLISH ACCESSORIES 44

How to Accessorize Chic and Stylish 45

How to Get Stylish Accessories 46

How to Make a Stylish Hair Accessory 47

What are the Basic Accessories that are Safe yet Stylish for Men? 48

Must Have Basic Accessories.. 49

CHAPTER 5: YOUR CROWNING GLORY 51

What Kinds of Hairstyles are Professional, Chic and Feminine? 51

What Kind of Hairstyle is Suitable for Students in High school?................... 54

What are Some Cute Hair Styles for a Scene/ Emo Chic? 55

How to Look Polished and Stylish with Very Long or Very Short Hair 55

Tips on How to Get Chic and Stylish Bangs 56

What is the Most Stylish Hair Cut for Your Face? 56

How can You Choose an Easy and Stylish Hair Cut? 57

CHAPTER 6: STYLING FEET 57

How to Look Stylish while Wearing Comfortable Shoes.......................... 58

Tips on Stylish Shoes for Casual Wearing 59

Styling Up a Cheap Pair of Shoes to Look Unique and Chic 61

Stylish and Comfortable Alternatives to Pumps 63

Choosing the Right Shoes for your Outfit 63

CHAPTER 7: STYLING UP THE TOES.............................65

Stylish Nail Designs 65

What Color of Nail Polish is Stylish?...67

Acrylic Nail Tips 67

Adding Style to Plain Black Nails 68

Stylish Nails with Art and Polish...68

CHAPTER 8: STYLE ON A BUDGET 69

How to Buy Stylish Clothing on a Budget 69

How to Make Old Clothes Look New and Stylish 71

How to Stylishly Use Your Old Accessories.......................................72

CHAPTER 9: CONCLUSION..72

Chapter 1: How to be Stylish and Chic

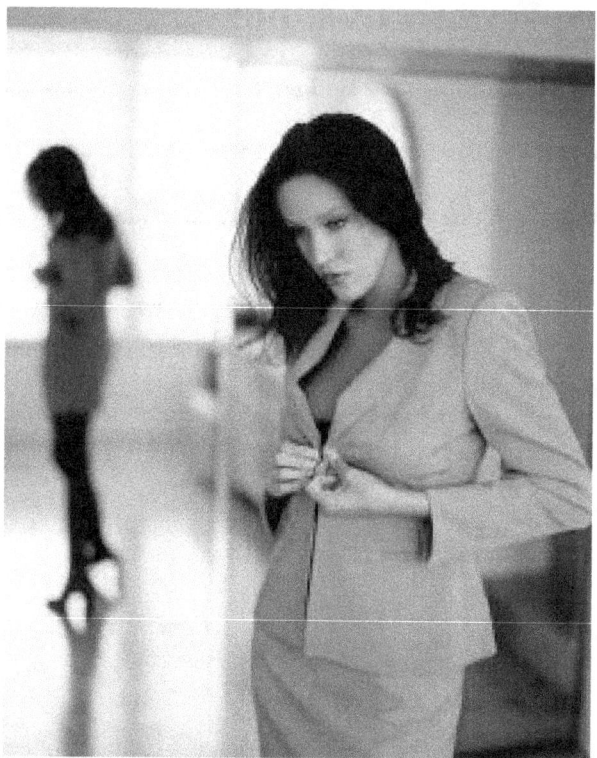

Introduction

When you get dressed before leaving your home every day, you probably take a couple of seconds to consider what you're going to wear. In doing so, you are subconsciously determining what you want the world to think about you. With your runners, ripped jeans, and faded concert t-shirt, the world may very well assume that you are hip, young, and don't care about fashion!

In many cases you are probably getting dressed for comfort and ease of wear for whatever you may be planning that day; a day at school, going out with friends, a lunch date, clubbing, a trip to the grocery store, or even just taking the dog for a walk. If you want to be perceived as being stylish and chic, but you thought that you had to sacrifice comfort, then worry no more! You can officially be chic, stylish, and comfortable in today's fashion world! You just have to know what you're doing!

When you hear the words "chic" and "stylish" do you think of snobby, preppy folks standing around a grand piano, drinking their cosmopolitans standing under a crystal chandelier? That is sometimes the image that is evoked, but chic and stylish fashion is much more accessible than that.

According to Wikapedia.com chic means: "stylish or smart, and is an element of fashion," while stylish means "having style; specifically: conforming to current fashion"

If you move into the world in your "Stylish Chic" dress code, you are really just moving about the world in "nice clothes" that are on trend. The stylish chic wardrobe does not include flip flops, torn clothes, or things that would not be acceptable in the middle class business world.

Fashion is a very personal expression and helps show your inner style to the world. It is fun and exciting to jump on board the hottest and latest trends with the change of every season, but not every style will appeal to you. Instead of jumping on the fashion bandwagon and reinventing yourself every season, focus on getting to know what you like and what looks good on you and add a couple of interesting pieces each season to highlight the trends instead of dressing yourself from head to toe in them.

Be true to your fashionable self and wear styles that make you feel good about how you look. That is the true essence of what is chic and stylish. The way you carry yourself will add confidence to your look and that is so very important in the world of fashion.

When you are following the trends that are outlined in this report remember that what matters more than what is the number one fashion piece of the day is how it makes you feel. If there is a piece of clothing from last year's collection that makes you feel like a million bucks, then by all means you should continue to wear it and add smaller touches to your wardrobe to keep it fresh.

What truly matters most in fashion is that you are comfortable with yourself. Love yourself and the world will love you. Second guess yourself and the world will see your lack of confidence, and no matter how stylish and chic you look, being less than self-assured will show in your posture, and the way you carry yourself.

A self-assured fashionable woman will stand tall with her shoulders back and not try to hide herself by slouching and hunching over. She will embrace her height or lack thereof, and look the world squarely in the eye while flashing a confidant smile that says: "look at me!"

Hopefully the tips outlined in this book will help you assemble a first rate wardrobe that will keep you on the fashion forward path.

Chapter 2: General Clothing Styles

There are hundreds upon hundreds of fashion magazines out there today both in print and online that can give you an idea of what is hot in the fashion world. Sometimes, however, the transition from the glossy pages of those magazines to the real world scenario isn't easy.

Many times these fashions are made only for the runway and could not possibly survive a transition to the street. Oftentimes these fashion pieces are an over the top artistic interpretation of what the designer wants to see.

Some designers are very down to earth and present shows full of fashion that you will be seeing walking down the street in the next couple of seasons, and sometimes you may just recognize elements of the show on the street. For example, while some designs may not be practical for the everyday woman, they may provide an inspiration for other designs, like the animal print trend that surfaced a few years back and is still going strong.

Other considerations when looking at these fashions forward examples is your own body shape. There are many people in the world who look like the models who are showing off the designs, but the bigger reality is that more of the world's population does not look like them.

How to Create the Stylish Look

It is important to know your body shape and to always pick clothing that will flatter your shape. Bodyshapeoffashion.com has an online calculator that will help you determine your body shape. Are you an apple, a pear, a strawberry, an hour glass, or rectangle? Styles that are flattering to an hourglass shape, and would highlight your waistline may not be the best options for a rectangular body shape.

Your goal when dressing to your body shape is to highlight your best assets and minimize those areas that you are not 100% in love with!

Another key factor when creating a stylish looks for yourself is to make sure that you are comfortable. Assess for yourself what that means to you and make sure that you strive for it in your clothing. If you are not someone who is comfortable with form fitting clothing that highlights all of your shape, then stay away from them, or find ways to incorporate them in a wardrobe that will make you comfortable. For example, if you do not like clothing that is clingy, then be sure to try on the clothing and adjust for sizes accordingly.

It is also important to keep an open mind when it comes to comfort. You may not know how it fits or feels until you have tried it on and lived in it for a few hours. Many times people who do not like form fitting fashion stay away from all clothing with any stretch to it. Fashion designers are incorporating Lycra into many items, from pants to socks, to shirts. They are not the traditional super tight fit that you may associate with spandex; in fact, the slights stretch they give may increase your comfort, especially in the waistbands of pants and skirts and move ability in shirts and tops.

In fashion, it is always a good idea to try to move outside your comfort zone with small pieces. If you are traditionally a very conservative dresser with many of your staple pieces being neutral, do not make that very huge leap and bring in very wild and vivid prints and colors on big items. You may be more comfortable if you make the leap to the animal print trend with a leopard print bangle or sunglasses instead of the zebra print blouse.

Keep your statement pieces under control, too! For example, with the animal print trend it can be tempting to add lots of pieces, but remember that less is more. One key piece in the animal print can give the impact you want. Too many pieces added together can make you look like a George of the Jungle wannabe.

That being said, you must always stay true to yourself. If you are someone who is more comfortable in flip flops and jeans, then suddenly transforming yourself into someone in dresses and sky high heels may not stick. Do not wear something if it feels like it isn't you! If you are not comfortable in the style of clothing you are wearing, it will show to everyone around you. And the biggest rule of fashion is to be confident. And you do not look confident at all if you are struggling with your spaghetti strap top or pulling down the hemline of your skirt.

When you are looking at stylish and chic pieces to add to your wardrobe be sure to purchase items that you like. It sounds silly and simple, but many times it happens that a shopper falls in love with an idea, but may not really like the piece they buy. For example, if you are on trend with the neon crazy right now, you may find yourself wanting to add in the electric hues with a new purse, but if you do not spend time examining the purse, you may get home with a bag in a color you love, but with absolutely no place for your cell phone or keys and limited functionality.

If you keep up with the latest trends, you will always have your finger on the pulse of what is chic and stylish. This will help you stay on top of what is current and what is not so that when you do go to add some new pieces to your wardrobe, you will know what is a good deal for you and what is only on sale because it is last year's style.

When you are putting together a chic and stylish look, it is a good idea to invest in accessories. Having on trend accessories can raise your last year styles to a current level and make the overall impact that you are looking for!

Earrings, bracelets, watches, belts, shoes, hats, purses, rings, and sunglasses should not be overlooked because they can all help to modernize your current wardrobe. They can add a trendy splash to your closet without breaking the bank, and you can do it while maintaining your comfort zone.

When you want to create your own chic and stylish look, it is very tempting to follow the masses to where the most popular items are sold, but resist the urge! Be creative and find the stores people are not flocking to so that you can find something that will be uniquely yours. That will help you avoid showing up a function where three other people are wearing the same outfit as you.

Don't discount the smaller independent shops. They are often very on trend and can offer you a different perception of the trend which will translate into a more individualized fashion pallet.

One final point on general style is to ensure that when you are shopping or just looking at your wardrobe you have items you love. You will need to make sure that you have outfits in your wardrobe. Items that you love are fantastic and will help give you that little pick me up you might need when getting dressed, but they can give the impression of being thrown together and not co-ordinating.

Having outfits at the ready, will ensure that you look put together and polished which are two very important factors in looking stylish and fashionable.

Becoming More Stylish

There are many ways to add some fashion flare to your wardrobe and to become more chic and stylish in your everyday wear: and most of the time it comes down to being aware.

If you have a very fashion forward friend or family member, then use them as a resource. Talk to them about what is hot right now and get their input. Perhaps they have a fashion blog that they follow religiously or a program or print magazine that they subscribe to. Use their knowledge and information to stay on trend.

Window shopping can be a very big help in determining what is stylish. Grab a friend and make a date to spend an afternoon wandering through your local mall or downtown center. If that's not your thing, then take a couple of hours and browse online and see what is happening in the world of fashion.

When you actually go to the store to window shop, you have the advantage of being able to see the clothing in person: to touch it and feel the fabric; and to see how it moves in real life; and you can actually try them on. These things can be very helpful in determining if they will make their way into your closet because the downfall of shopping online or from a catalogue has always been that you don't know how they feel until you get them and try them on.

Media is everywhere and is a fantastic source of information on what is chic and stylish? Pay attention to the free opinions that are swirling around out there! Magazines, fashion blogs, television shows, awards coverage, and dedicated networks like the fashion channel will absolutely give you an idea of what is front and center in the fashion world today?

Attending local events is another great way to see what is happening in fashion. If you attend a social function, then you will see what other people are wearing. It is an added bonus to see these fashion pieces out in the world and to get an idea of how they work in real life. You can see what works and what does not work and get a very good impression of it would fit into your lifestyle.

Take advantage of "public services" in your community that will help you get on the right track. Some organizations offer workshops and wardrobe building sessions that are free or of very low cost that can offer you some suggestions and guidance in this area.

Did you know that there are people in the world who get paid to do just this? Personal shoppers are available at a cost in most high end department stores. They will assess your shape and size and get a feel for what colors and fabrics you favor and then they will set up regular meetings with you to show you what has come into their store that fits your bill.

Some stores that do not have a personal shopper department may have some very informed and educated sales people on site who can do the same thing for you without the fee. Many smaller shops have staff on site who are very astute and can make fantastic suggestions to help you update your wardrobe.

If it is not in your budget to hire a professional, then become your own best professional! Spend some time reflecting on what you like and what you do not like; weed out your closet and find items that are your favorites, and determine why. Is it because of how they fit, the color, or just how they make you feel when you wear them?

Get to know what you like and create an inspiration board for yourself. Pin up pictures of colors, fabric samples, patterns, pieces you like, whatever you see in a magazine, online, or just something you have snapped a picture of, and look for similar themes.

Keep your mind open and make a conscious effort to move outside your comfort zone, but do it in a safe way. Don't make huge leaps away from your wardrobe staples unless you are ready for that! Take small steps and watch the huge impact they have on your fashion sense!

How Do You Dress Up in a Chic and Stylish Way?

Keeping a neutral pallet on hand gives you great starting place for your wardrobe.

Everyone should have neutral bottoms in their closet. Neutrals generally include black or beige and sometimes navy. Pants in any of these colors that are well maintained, fit beautifully and are comfortable to wear are a must! Ladies may include a skirt, if you are skirt wearers, in a tailored comfortable length.

Dark denim in any fit is also considered a staple. You can get tones of mileage out of your denim if you care for it properly, so choose wisely; it could be with you for a while!

A crisp white (or off white) button down shirt in a classic fit is another wardrobe staple that everyone should have. This can easily be dressed up and down with your trendy pieces depending on what you want to do with them.

When you have the basics already, you can add trendy pieces to your wardrobe and update your style with the seasons for a much lower price than re-hauling it every time the trends change.

If you are aware of the trends out there and know how you feel about them, then you will very easily be able to determine what you would like to incorporate into your wardrobe. Pick items that are on trend and that will move with you from this season into the next one. It is not important to hold on trend item any longer than that. They will most likely have run their course any longer than that. So budget accordingly. If a fashion piece's lifespan is only about six months, then determine how much you are willing to spend on it in comparison to the other pieces in your wardrobe.

When you pick items, be very aware of the fit and your body shape. Pencil skirts are very popular right now, but not every figure is comfortable wearing them. The same goes for cigarette pants and skinny jeans. Both are very on trend right now, but not everybody's shape may feel comfortable wearing them.

Take the time to try on the items you are considering and make sure that they fit properly. No matter how stylish or chic the item is, if it does not fit you properly and you are not comfortable wearing it, you will not get your money's worth out of it.

Keep the colors in your basics neutral, as mentioned before. Black and white is elegant and chic. That color combination can transcend all seasons and styles. It will also give you a great background to highlight your new "must have" pieces with lots of colors and patterns.

Fashion is becoming less about the clothes and more and more about how you feel. Fashion should be an extension of you, so find the clothes you love and wear the attitude you want to world to see!

How Do You Choose Trendy Fashionable Clothes Ideally Suited for You?

Finding clothes that are on trend and suited for you can be a bigger challenge than it appears. Oftentimes the fashions are targeted for individuals under a certain age, and it can be very uncomfortable for everyone to see people in a much higher age bracket wearing them!

Dress your age. It is a relatively simple theory in fashion, but it can be harder than you would first suspect. Trends are not directed by age, but fashion can be.

For example, the skin tight micro mini in leopard prints may be made for the 20's something clubbing crowd. That does not mean that people in their 30s and over cannot and should not join the trend. The animal prints trend has moved across many areas and can be found almost everywhere.

Know what works for you and your lifestyle and what does not. If you are a business professional in your 40s, the skin tight neon leggings that are back in fashion today might not work for you in your everyday business life, but a surprising shock of color in your accessories or a pretty pop of neon layered into your outfit may work very well for you.

When you are choosing fashions to wear, select one asset to highlight and focus on it! Many people fall into the trap of highlighting too many assets and their outfit which could have been very chic and stylish suddenly looks trashy and cheap.

For women, the obvious areas to highlight are cleavage, legs, back, waist, arms, and neck. However, if someone was to try to showcase all of these areas in one outfit, it may seem that she was wearing very little at all, and while skin can be sexy, too much skin can very quickly turn sleazy. Each outfit you choose can highlight a different asset to make the most of your wardrobe and your attributes!

When you are shopping for trendy clothes get out of the house and off line and go to the store and try them on; it really is the only way you can determine if it is a good fit for you.

Take suggestions from the people working in the store and ask them for suggestions. You will not have to purchase them, but it's a good idea to get another person's perspective on fashion and what might look good on you because we tend to fall into our own subconscious patterns. Take a look in your own closet. Odds are you will quickly find a trend in the items you already have, either in color, cut, or style. Another person's perspective may bring some needed color or flair to your wardrobe.

When all else fails, get some professional help! Talk to people who work in fashion. Look for a body image consultant or personal shopper. Find out what will look good on you and get some suggestions for styles, then start trying them on and determining for yourself what looks and feels good.

Remember when you are shopping and enlisting help, suggestions are just that. Suggestions from a professional do not mean that you now have to buy it even if you hate it. It just means that you are open to finding a new and fresh perspective on what might work for you!

What are the Key Pieces in a Chic and Stylish Wardrobe?

When you are dressing you should consider your clothing to be like a building. The first thing you will need to consider is your foundation. This is equally important for both men and women.

Experts say that nearly 70% of women are wearing the wrong size bra, and more than 90% are wearing a style that is not right for them. Wearing the wrong size and style of bra can dramatically affect how your clothing fits and feels which can bang how you feel in your clothes!

Many lingerie and department stores have bra fitters on site and offer a complimentary bra fitting to their customers. It is suggested that your bra should be re-sized every six months due to changes in your body shape.

A good fitting bra will not pinch anywhere, the straps will stay put, and the back strap will not ride up your back. In addition, your breasts will remain covered and will not spill out of your cups.

Wearing the right colored bra will also help you create a more polished and stylish look. It is suggested that you refrain from wearing black or white bras and select fabrics that more closely match the color of your skin. No matter what the trend or fashion of the moment, it is generally accepted that wearing a colored or patterned bra with a white t-shirt is not fashionable or sexy.

Consider the fashions you will be wearing and purchase undergarments accordingly. If you prefer the lighter, more form fitting t-shirt materials that are out there right now, then consider purchasing a t-shirt bra which provides more coverage.

The lumps and bumps created by wearing the wrong size and style of bra can dramatically affect your profile. Wearing the right bra can trim about 10 pounds off of your silhouette, and in this world of fashion, who wouldn't want to shave a few extra pounds?

Undergarments like briefs and panties must also be considered. It is important to match your briefs and panties to the clothing you are wearing. For example, if you are wearing white or light beige colored pants, skirts, or shorts, then avoid the dark colored or patterned under things. The color will show through your pants and not offer a very polished or chic look.

Panty lines are not fashionable or chic either, so be aware of the cut and fabric in your bottoms and dress accordingly. Likewise, it is not considered fashionable or chic to display your "t-bar" over the top of your pants when you bend down. So if you are wearing a thong, then make sure your top is long enough to cover what may show up!

Once you have built your foundation then start looking at ways to dress up the rest of your wardrobe. There are staples that everyone should have in their wardrobe. If you don't already have these, then start here before adding the more trendy pieces.

As mentioned before, keep your basics neutral: bottoms that are black, beige or navy, dark skirt in a flattering style and fit and dark denims.

Depending on what you do for a living, you may find that having dark washed denim in a flattering cut and fit is of the utmost importance. They have found their place in many corporate cultures on more than just "casual Fridays". Many cuts and styles of dark denim have been incorporated into the dress list of work. There are many styles and cuts available today from boot cut to relax, to fit, and to slim leg, so try them on and find the fit that works for you.

Be sure that they are comfortable, provide good coverage of your assets, and will move with you throughout the day.

Having layering pieces is always a good idea to help your transition from season to season and day to night. Cashmere is always in style and provides a lightweight option to help you cover up at work, out with friends and just about anywhere. Pick up a light weight cardigan in a staple color like black or white for longevity, and in hot trendy colors to instantly update your regular wardrobe.

Every woman should have at least one pair of black pants that are not denim in her closet that she can go to when jeans just won't cut it. They need to be in a flattering cut and ones that make her feel comfortable and confident. These black pants can be instantly dressed up with a sparkly top and heels or down with a button down and ballet flats to fit any occasion.

They can be pulled out in a pinch for a job interview, to meet the dean of the college or other important business contact, or for a more stylish night out with friends or a partner. Be sure that you love them because you will be spending lots of time together! You can never go wrong with your go to black pants.

The little black dress or LBD which was made famous by Audrey Hepburn in "Breakfast at Tiffany's" is another invaluable article that every woman should have at her disposal. The best LBD to have will be the one that makes you feel strong, sexy, and confident every time you put it on.

There are many different styles of LBD to look at and consider. Many are a shorter length, falling just above the knee, to the knee. This is a length of skirt that looks good on most women; it is sexy enough to show off some leg, but not too sexy so as to show off everything else!

Some LBD have very sexy and stylish cut with shorter length, more dramatic neckline, and possibly an interesting back. Others are very classically cut in a straight shift dress styling. Some have sleeves, some do not. Some come with interesting and decorative embroidery or bead work, while others are very simple. If it is a timeless piece, like a straight shift dress then it will grow and live on with every fashion re-incarnation and can be quickly put on trend with the appropriate accessories.

Day to day styling is where you spend most of your time so it is also where you need to focus most of your attention. It is important to find the right shoes to compliment your special occasion outfit, and it will be discussed, but it is even more important to find the comfortable and stylish shoes that will take you from the subway to the office, across campus, to the meeting, and out with friends every day.

There are women in the world who seem to have been made for 4" heels. There are many more who are not. While your converse all-stars may be the most comfortable shoes you have ever worn, they will not help you move from office to dinner party. Take the time to try on and investigate the biggest season trend for the last few years: The ballet flat. Comfortable, stylish flats will help keep your toes in great form while you still put out a tailored and polished look.

Having an "of the moment" bag or clutch can immediately elevate your jeans and tunic top to an awards show worthy prize! These bags can bring an element of functionality to your wardrobe as well which makes them a great investment of your time and money!

Another key piece to keep in your fashion arsenal is a pair of good fitting comfortable khaki pants. There are many styles that are hot right now, like the ever-popular cargo pocket khaki pants that will take you effortlessly from one casual gathering to another.

Khaki is another neutral shade that can complement many of your fashionable separates and the lighter color is certainly more seasonally appropriate for the hotter weather than the dark neutrals like black, navy, brown and even charcoal.

Khaki's refer to the color as opposed to the style of the pants. Khakis took on their first life in the military inspired styles of the late 1980s and early 1990s. They gained popularity and held fast in a variety of cuts and styles. In a fashion timeline, it would appear that khaki pants have been on the radar forever, which as you know in fashion speak, is a very long time!

Today khaki's can refer to the traditional long cargo style pant, which is very casual; the khaki cargo skirt or Capri pant; or other comfortable, trendy fits like boot cut, slim fit, or relaxed fit which will suit your lifestyle and carry you from the office to a casual dinner out with friends.

Because khakis come in so many different cuts and styles there is one out there that is perfect for you. Perhaps it is the traditional relaxed fit style that goes so nicely with your preferred button down styling. Perhaps it is the slim cut fit that really flows with your equestrian style riding boots. Or maybe it is even the city short length khakis that make your summer style effortless at work.

Khakis, depending on the cut and the style, will fit into your wardrobe and help you rock today's hottest styles and trends whether it be bold infusions of color, sky high heels, super skinny belts or oversized fashion bags. The old faithful khaki pants are comfortable in all of these situations and more. Make them your next must have item to buy!

One of the final suggestions of key pieces to have in your stylish and chic wardrobe is something that may only be viewed by you or a close friend or two, but its importance is huge.

If you are committed to dressing stylishly and fashionably, then you cannot let it end when you go home to relax.

In order to keep your chic and stylish mind set keep your fashions chic and stylish no matter what you are doing. Sleeping in faded plaid boxer shorts and an old college t-shirt certainly is comfortable and can feel like a second skin, but it is not the fashionable mindset that you want to wake up in every morning.

Pajamas have come a long way from the flannel menswear inspired sets of years gone by. They also have grown to include more than a silk slip style. Fashionable and trendy pajamas today include chic and comfortable sleep pants in pant, short and Capri lengths. The materials used in these Jammies will help you keep your elegant and stylish feel. Many of them use the ultra soft jersey material, silk, satin, and other cosy materials.

The tops are as varied as the bottoms and can include tank tops with build in support, snug fitting long sleeved t-shirts, cover ups, and wrap housecoats. These ensembles will help you keep your fashionable and chic appearance and mindset no matter what you're doing at home. And when you find a set that you love, you will be amazed at how comfortable they are. You won't even notice that you're not wearing your Michigan State t-shirt!

With the many different styles out there that are fashions forward like Hobo bags, slings, clutches, and micro minis, you are bound to be able to find one that works with your lifestyle!

Chapter 3: Stylish Dressing

Fashion awareness is happening earlier and earlier for kids today. Starting as early as the age of 2, some children demand a hand in determining their fashion statement each day. Once they hit about the age of eight, many moms and dads are getting involved in lengthy battles with their children over what is acceptable and not acceptable on the fashion front. Some parents choose to fight through this front while others take the opportunity to educate their children on fashion and what it really means, which can help alleviate some headaches in the future.

Tips on How to Dress Like a Stylish Teen

Adolescence is the greatest time in a woman's fashion history! She is young, probably in the best shape of her life, and does not yet have to conform to any set standard. She does not have a job that requires her to dress a certain way. She is expected and sometimes encouraged to experiment with her fashion at this stage to help her determine who she really is.

There are many "teen" trends that have remained on the screen for decades. These are not necessarily the "trendy" fashions, but ones that are there. Gothic dressing, which incorporates a lot of black clothing, white or pale make up and dark hair styling's have been very common place for years, while punk styling, which includes lots of color, high hair, and interesting accessories has come and gone.

The teen years are a time of experimentation with appearance. Sometimes it is done for the shock factor and other times it is done out of a genuine desire to explore and understand other people's experiences.

Stylish teens today tend to steer away from the gothic and punk interpretations and embrace the essence of a carefree youth.

The uniform of a trendy and stylish teen today includes lots of fitted clothing, cute shirts, shoes, accessories and hair and makeup in bright vivid colors.

Fitted clothing like jeggings, tights, or skinny jeans are a staple in the trendy teen's closet. She has them in multiple colors and patterns, and wears them for many different occasions. She balances these super fitted items with the larger, and sometimes oversized, cute shirts with iconic images, interesting patterns, and quotes or popular culture references.

Color is probably the biggest trend in teen styles today. Neon colors are bright and popular and can be seen everywhere on teens from sunglasses to backpacks, to cell phone cases, and nail polish.

Fashion and clothing are such a personal expression, especially for teens.

How Can You Look Really Stylish and Chic at Prom?

Prom is unmistakably one of the biggest social events in high school for a teen. Proms have achieved an almost fairy tale status in today's society with so much attention being given by Hollywood in movies and on Television. Every girl deserves to feel like Cinderella at her prom! Regardless of the ideologies around prom, one thing remains front and center, the prom dress.

The key to looking chic and stylish at prom is to be original. When you are shopping for a prom dress, be realistic about what you want. Trends change regularly when it comes to color, length, and style of dresses, but what is most important is how you feel about your dress.

If the trends are leaning towards super short, one shouldered pastel dresses and your dream has always been to dance at your prom in a ball gown length hot pink number with a sweet heart neckline, then go for it! There are many off the rack options for you to consider when looking for dresses that will be very trendy, but if it is within the budget, then there are always tailor made options as well.

Make sure that your dress is fun! That means a couple of different things. Be comfortable in your dress. It is no fun trying to dance with one hand holding up the front of your dress and the other hand pulling down the back. It is also not much fun to have to sit out your entire night because your dress keeps knocking people over. Make sure that your dress allows you to have fun.

Prom is a celebration: it's the end of high school and the start of your "grown up" life. Make sure that your dress gives off a fun vibe. It is not a funeral, it's a party! So be sure that your dress captures how you feel about this momentous event in your life.

Your dress needs to be flattering. Be realistic when you go dress shopping. How it looks on the mannequin at the front of the store does not indicate how it will look on you. Try it on and move in it. If it slips and slides or pinches and tugs then it might not be the right style for you. While it's always a good idea to have an idea of what you're looking for, it is also equally important to have an open mind.

Be sure that the dress you choose will compliment your body shape and will not fight against it all night. Your goal is to look good, feel great, and more importantly, have an amazing time at your prom, so pick a dress that will allow you to do that.

This season, color is huge. Soft muted colors are very last year. The trendiest of teens will be wearing frocks in bright, strong colors.

How to Dress Stylish in College

When you are in college your attention is usually focused more on assignments, exams, and what you are going to do after graduation! The traditional costume of the college student includes sweatpants, school spirit hoods, and UGGs: all things that scream comfort, but things that do not always project the stylish, chic image you are hoping to cultivate.

Determining where you stand on a fashion front as a college student is a huge task. You may not feel that you are "ready" to take on a professional wardrobe and may fall victim to the "comfort means fashion suicide" mentality of a student.

Fashion on a college student's budget is not easy to do. When you find pieces to buy, you know that they have to be worth the investment in order for it to make sense financially for you. While it may be true that you can buy two pairs of sweatpants for the cost of one pair of nicely tailored, well fit dark denim pants, you will be able to wear those jeans differently and to more places than your sweats will allow.

School spirit is a wonderful thing, but if all of your t-shirts and sweaters have school logos on them, then odds are you are not putting on the stylish and chic face you may have hoped you were.

Comfort does not have to be sacrificed for fashion. If you like the warmth of the fleece lined hood, you can find the same feel with a more fashion forward face with a jersey knit shirt and cardigan.

Bright colors and fresh prints are huge on campuses today. They provide a fashionable chic look while still embracing your youth. Abstract prints are making a huge impact today and provide great mixing abilities with a variety of colors and styles.

Combining casual and formal pieces that you already have can give you a very polished look on campus. Black dress pants with a cool abstract print t-shirt can give you the balance you need in your wardrobe.

UGG boots and flip flops are comfortable and practical, but they do not give you a polished looks. Look for sandals that are pretty as well as practical that can lend an air of elegance to your outfit. And consider how much more refined a pair of riding boots would look with your skinny jeans than your UGGs do.

When President Barack Obama delivered his commencement address at Barnard College in New York City this year, he shared with the graduating class that his wife Michelle Obama has taught women that "you can be stylish and powerful too".

What to Wear on a Company Dinner?

In the work world you know that you need to be prepared for just about anything. A regular day of work can quickly be extended to an evening of dinner meetings or entertaining out of town clients and your wardrobe needs to be flexible enough to do both at the drop of a hat.

Business dressing dictates a certain standard of decorum and that should be followed even when attending a company dinner. In order for you to project your professional image, you need to remain professional looking and you can absolutely do that in a fun and fashion forward way.

The general rule of thumb for professional dressing involves the three B's: No butts, no boobs, and no bellies.

Make sure that you are not showing too much cleavage at your company dinner. While you are officially off the clock, what happens at your corporate event will reflect back on you at work. Your company dinner may not be the right time for you to show off your newest high fashion treasure if it involves a plunging neckline or back.

Make sure that your "assets" are covered no matter what you are wearing. A too short skirt or peek-a-boo t-bar from your lime green thong will not allow your employer to keep a professional image of you in their mind.

Unless you are a professional belly dancer, fitness trainer, or waitress at Hooters® showing your belly for any work function is not acceptable. It is not stylish to see that much skin and it is certainly not a professional look.

Keep your basics in mind when dressing for a company dinner and remember that you goal is to look polished and professional while allowing your after hours style to shine through a bit.

This may be a great opportunity for you to wear colors or patterns that you might not be able to wear at work. For example, wearing a black skirt (or dress pants) with an embellished neon pink tank and flyaway black cardigan might be perfectly professional and on trend enough for you to feel comfortable at your after hours business event.

Putting together a chic and stylish outfit for your professional event is as important as the outfit you put together for work each day. Allow your personality and style sense to shine through, and keep the focus on you, and not just your assets.

Remember this is a business outing and not a night out clubbing with your friends. It is important that you dress in a way that is comfortable for you while not making those around you uncomfortable. Chic and stylish does not necessarily mean sexy, especially at work function!

How to Dress Stylishly in Plus-Sized Clothing

Today's fashion markets are not as unevenly divided as they once were. There was a time when anyone who wore above a size 10 would not be able to secure any fashionable clothes for herself. Thankfully, with the development of high end plus size retailers and the integration of plus sized models into the fashion industry curvy women can dress as fashionably as their petite counterparts.

When dressing a plus sized figure, be sure to pay attention to cuts, styles and fabrics. You want to dress to flatter your figure and highlight your best attributes, not draw attention to the areas of your body you'd prefer to down play.

Fabric can play a very big role. Some fabrics are not very forgiving and will highlight bulges and rolls, while others are very flattering and will support and smooth your figure giving you a tremendous silhouette.

Patterns can be your best friend or they can quickly turn into your worst enemy in plus sized fashion. Patterns that look sweet and cute on a size two mini skirt can quickly overwhelm the senses in a sized 16 version. Incorporate patterns sparingly and use them as an accent piece, not as a building basis.

The reason that patterns can turn into your enemy is that they are an optical illusion that can change the way that people see you.

For example, if you are wearing an item with horizontal lines (going from side to side), those lines pull the eye with them causing every eye to see you from one side to the other. This can make you appear wider around than you are because of the way it plays on your eyes. Likewise, if you are wearing vertical stripes (going up and down), it will make you appear longer and leaner because the eye is moving up and down, not side to side.

Do not be frightened by this because you can still wear horizontal stripes very successfully. To successfully wear horizontal stripes, be sure that the stripe print is small. Smaller, darker, more plentiful stripes will keep the eyes moving from side to side quickly. Wider, lighter stripes will allow the eyes to linger on the line which could make you appear thicker. Today's nautical inspired stripes are a great example of good stripes. Many are backed on a black or navy blue background and include a very thin white stripe.

Don't underestimate the power of black. Dark clothing can work as a slimming agent. But don't be sold on only black. Wear a darker color to anchor your outfit, like black, navy, brown, or charcoal and pair it with a colorful, fun top. While it is important to keep the bottoms anchored in dark colors, you are not in mourning; you're just trying to elongate your look!

A curious addition to the styles you already know and love is the re-occurrence of the popularity of the wide leg pants. Menswear inspired pants are all the rage this year and they do wonders for the plus sized figure. You may be questioning how bigger pants can make you look more sleek, but it is true. A wide leg pant will help you create the illusion of a straight line from top to bottom which will help to smooth out any other bumps and lumps that you might want to flatten.

Whatever the style of pants, skirt or Capri's you may be wearing, be sure that they are long enough. While there isn't really a correct answer to how long your bottoms should be, it is certainly worth taking a second to eyeball where they end. Pants, Capri's, and skirts should end where you want people to look. So ideally, they would end at the most shapely point of your legs. If, however, they end at a wider or unpolished part of your leg, they can end up cutting your legs off too short which in turn makes them look stubby.

Another elegant trick of dressing is to embrace the pointed toe shoes. You may ask why, but it is quite simple really. A pointed toe at the end of an elongated leg will visually help to elongate the legs even further by keeping the eye moves down the leg to the end of the toe, and then to a sharp point. By contrast, rounded toe shoes make the legs look frumpy and end the leg abruptly.

The fabric that your bottoms are made of can make or break the entire outfit. If you choose loose flowing materials, it can add extra bulk to your outfit and may not be the flattering silhouette you are searching for. Likewise, super clingy material may not be the most flattering. The idea fabric will allow the clothing to skim over your body, not cling to it. Your pants and skirts and Capris should move like a second skin, and ideally, you shouldn't give them a second thought once you put them on.

Finally, one last tip when you are shopping for stylish and chic bottoms. Back pockets are a must. They visually break-up the material on your seat and put it into a different proportion. Be aware that small pockets or ones that are too small for the area they are on will make your butt look big. Bigger pockets can help to visually reduce the size of your seat. Balance out the size of the pockets with the size of the seat.

Layering Clothes in a Stylish Way

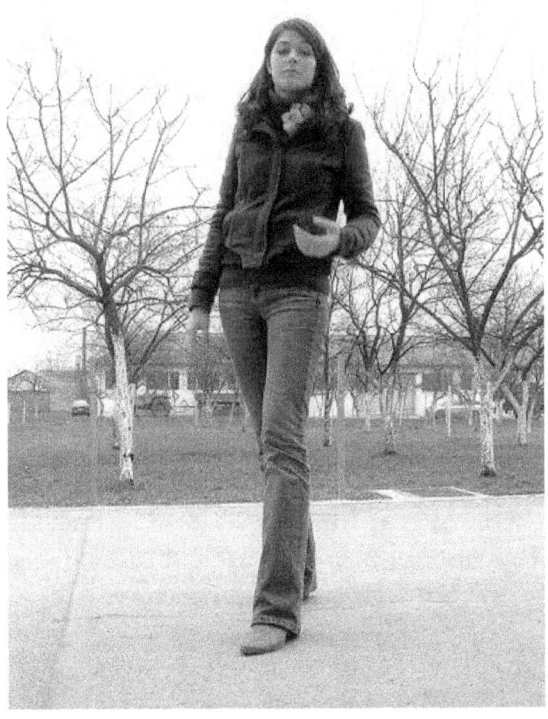

Layering your clothes is a style that many people associate with the colder months of the year, but it is something that can be done successfully in all seasons, and can help keep your wardrobe fresh.

When you are layering your clothing, go for style, not bulk. While there is no hard and fast rule of how to go about doing it, it is a general rule of thumb to never layer more than four distinct pieces. More than three moves you from stylish and chic to looking like your cold.

In layering, you will want to start from the inside of the outfit and move outwards. Generally speaking you will want to include the lightest layers closest to your skin and move on to the heaviest layers on the top. For example, you would not want to start with a heavy wool sweater and then layer a lace blouse over top. It would make the most sense to start with the lace blouse and then add the wool sweater with the delicate poufs of lace showing through.

Another geographic point to remember is that the longest pieces should stay towards the bottom of the outfit. A long flowing cardigan should not be put over top of a cropped vest.

It is a good and safe opportunity to experiment with styles and patterns that you may not be comfortable enough to wear on their own. For example, if you are not sure you can pull off the ultra girly ruffle top, it might be a "safer" bet for you to wear it under a more structured vest to make it feel more comfortable for you.

When you are layering pieces, it is important to take note and only include one focal piece. Do not allow your layers to compete with each other. For example, if you are incorporating the ruffle blouse, do not layer it with a ruffled edge cardigan. It will become overwhelming to your outfit.

Those are the basic rules of thumb. But other than that; the door is wide open! Think about mixing formal and casual pieces to maximize your wardrobe and keep your outfit balanced.

The obvious example would be wearing very stylish and chic high heels with your skinny jeans, but you can also wear your ruffled blouse with a jersey knit cardigan, or black leather vest. Contrast your layers for an interesting and exciting surprise!

This season, color is huge: the brighter the better. Use bold colors to play up your neutral layers. Think a pop of cobalt blue under layers of back, or a hot pink belt with your beige cardigan.

Sometimes when you are wearing layers you may be afraid of overwhelming your style with too many options. Do not allow that fear to stop you from adding an interesting second dimension to your outfit: Scarves, belts and accessories.

If they are bold statement pieces and you are not sure what to do, then play conservatively and leave it at one or two pieces, but if you love the look, then add as many key pieces as you like.

The challenge with layering fashions is to keep it light and fresh. Do not allow your frame to be overwhelmed with layers. You can quickly go from looking stylish to looking like you are playing dress up in your mother's closet. Resist the urge to overdress. In some cases, less really is more!

How to Find Trendy and Stylish Maternity Clothes

Women who are expecting today are among the luckiest pregnant women in history! Society has made huge medical advances in prenatal and post natal care, there are tons of convenient items that are getting greener and more accessible, and maternity fashions are stylish, chic and no longer consist of huge tenting fabric.

Today, chic and stylish maternity clothing is very easy to find. Most large department stores carry at least a small collection, and the speciality stores like Thyme and Motherhood are popping up all over the map.

We are very lucky to be in a season of style that is accommodating to maternity styles. If you look through the maternity racks in your local department store, you may be surprised to find that many of the hottest styles of the day are echoed in maternity styles, such as empire waist dresses, tunic tops, and skinny pants. The one trend colors and patterns are also being mirrored in the maternity departments much to the expectant mother's joy!

When you are dressing your chic and stylish baby bump, look to the masses of expectant celebrity mothers to see how to do it with class. Jessica Simpson, for example, even with her large baby weight gain, maintained her style and class throughout her nine months of pregnancy.

You can keep wearing your old clothes until they don't fit anymore and then switch to sweat or your partner's stuff, but if that is not the image you are hoping to portray, then get yourself to the store!

When you are dressing your bump, consider these guidelines to help your transition from regular to maternity clothes.

Your body will be growing and changing and for some women that can be a huge source of stress, especially when they're regular clothes no longer fit them. Remember that this is all happening for a good reason and you will soon be back in your pre-baby clothes. In the meantime, pick fashions and styles that draw the attention upwards to your face.

Wearing styles that focus the eye on your middle, (for example, the nautical stripes), will make you will appear larger than you actually are. If, however, you choose vertical stripes or interesting prints on your tops then you will automatically bring the eye upwards to your face, which, by the way, will be glowing.

Fitted styles may take some getting used to if that is not your normal style. They are very flattering to the expectant mom and can really highlight your growing baby bump.

Many maternity styles favor draping and criss-cross styling that will not only help emphasis your growing assets, but will add style and interest to your fashions.

Because your pregnancy will transcend at least three seasons you may want to get some "staple" pieces. Keep your basics and dresses dark to streamline your wardrobe and look chic. You can add in fashionable accents with jewellery, bags, and shoes to keep your looks on trend.

When you are expecting, there will be enough stresses in your life with the great changes about to occur. This may not be the time to experiment with a whole new style, or you may find that this is the perfect time to reinvent yourself. Whether you choose to reinvent yourself or keep your closets status quo remember to remain true to yourself.

Depending on your size fluctuations in pregnancy, you may be able to extend the life of your current wardrobe a little longer to help you maintain your chic and stylish wardrobe.

Baby bands are a spandex band that can be slipped on over your pants. They come in many designer colors and mimic the look of layering a long t-shirt under your tops. They are widely available at most maternity stores and are quite reasonably priced.

Knowing your body shape and being aware of how it changes through pregnancy will help you keep stylish throughout. If you are becoming more of an apple shape than your previous pear, you may want to consider keeping your dresses short because the long flowing maxi dresses that are popular right now may overwhelm your figure.

You may want to include the following items in your chic and stylish maternity wardrobe.

The foundation pieces are very important. Wearing a good bra throughout your pregnancy can prevent some of the unfortunate changes that may have otherwise occurred. In addition, a good comfortable bra will help you maintain your silhouette and keep everyone comfortable.

Maternity bras are also very widely sold in fashionable matching bra and panty sets. Remember that maternity wear does not have to be matronly wear! You can be the stylish, sexy, mama that you want to be.

Long, fitted t-shirts in a variety of popular colors are a great addition to your attire. They can easily be layered into other outfits and can keep be accessorized with jewellery, scarves, and cardigans.

Empire waist dresses are an obvious asset to the expectant mother. The high waist emphasises your bust line and allows the fabric to flow over your expanding middle. Stylish, chic and comfortable, especially when you purchase this style in the ever-popular jersey knit fabric in one of the season's hot colors.

Stylish and chic shoes are the pregnant woman's best friends when she strays away from the heels and buys them in the "flats" aisle. Many of the celebrity moms of today are being seen out on the town in sky high heels. For the average expectant mother, however, this can cause some distress on her feet and an aching lower back. Comfortable, trendy, stylish flats are a great addition to your maternity wardrobe and can be found in many hot colors as well as styles.

Who Says New Moms can't be Stylish and Chic?

Being a new mom can be a big adjustment in your life. Sometimes it is hard to realize that you are no longer just responsible for yourself; that this new little life is depending entirely on you for their survival; that you are someone's mom. Just because you are someone's mom doesn't mean that you have to start dressing like one! Today's mom can be a stylish and chic fashion plate.

When dressing as a new mom good foundation garments are important. This means not only wearing a good supportive bra that fits properly, but it can also include body shapers.

Oprah Winfrey popularized the Spanx® brand on her show when told the world that she wore them. There are many other brands out there as well, from high end to bargain basement and they will all work a little differently, so educate yourself about them.

Some body shapers are big, involved garments that include eye hooks, snaps, and zippers, not unlike the corsets of the Victorian era; while others are spandex, stretchy and require much less hardware.

The job of shape wear is to help smooth your silhouette and iron out the bumps. These little secrets can help you get back into your stylish pre-baby wardrobe quicker than you could ever imagine.

Another additional benefit of body shapers and other supportive undergarments is that in addition to helping you regain your stylish edge, they can help support your body to heal quickly following delivery. They can add addition support to otherwise weakened and tired abdominal muscles improving your posture and overall look.

Smart moms know that camouflage is importing in dressing stylishly after baby. Wearing on trend patterns can significantly reduce your anxiety when leaving the house after holding your baby; it can help hide stains and other faux pas inflicted on you by baby.

Breast feeding moms can remain stylish and chic when they are dressing with new lines of breastfeeding wear that is designed to look fantastic and still be very functional. Wrap dresses and tops are two items that are very smart to have at your disposal. Many fashion designers are now catering to the breastfeeding crowd, such as Milk Smart Mama.

Tunic tops and other light airy styles that are on trend right now are a very smart and stylish way to help you transition your wardrobe from pregnancy to new mom. The generously cut fabric will help you remain comfortable in the style while still allowing you to embrace the current trends.

Comfort is a key for the stylish and chic new mom. You never know when you will be called upon to feed on demand or contort yourself into interesting new shapes in order to change your baby in a non-baby friendly environment. For that reason, it is important to be comfortable when you are dressing.

Elastic waist and other stretch waist pants were never considered fashionable or stylish, but thankfully now, many major retailers are bringing in these styles en masse. It is not uncommon to find stylish and chic pencil skirts at general retailers with a "comfort fit" waistband which allows you to pull on the item for a perfect fit.

Wearing high heels as a new mom coupled with the lack of sleep you are experiencing compounded by your body that is re-balancing itself after childbirth can bring disaster to a new mom. Invest in good quality, comfortable flat shoes that will mix and match with your wardrobe so that leaving the house will be effortless, at least when it comes to your shoes. Embellished ballet flats in a variety of colors and menswear inspired oxford flats are two of the biggest trends in footwear right now.

Nursing tank tops used to be pretty noticeable on the racks in the store as well as on the new mom. Today however, they go virtually unnoticed among the "regular" tops. Finding these staple pieces that you can use to layer your wardrobe will allow you flexibility and comfort in your attire: two things that every mom will definitely want more of!

Investing in a good pair of dark, well-tailored jeans will be an asset to your wardrobe. As mentioned before, it is a good staple piece that can be dressed up or down. Finding a comfortable pair that holds you and hugs you in all the right places can certainly go in your favor and make you feel supported and beautiful. It is that confidence that can help you carry off any style!

Being a mom doesn't mean that you have to give up your cool handbags in favor of an unfashionable diaper bag or backpack. Many high end retailers are marketing their baby friendly products to moms who want to remain chic and stylish with baby on their hips. Many high end purse lines offer a diaper bag option. There is also a "diaper bag insert" on the market which will allow you to transform your favorite fashionable bag into a functional diaper bag that will still look amazing, and far better than that quilted ducky bag you saw.

In the closets of very fashionable new moms you will likely find some very stylish "cover ups". Swing cardigans (the kinds that don't actually do up) are wonderful additions to your wardrobe. They offer a very "now" way to dress up your more casual clothing and take you from around the house to running errands in style.

Swing cardigans are usually found in the hip brushing length, which is great for hiding figure flaws including those last few baby pounds you may still be carrying with you. Pick cardigans in fresh, now colors and hot new patterns to keep your wardrobe on trend.

Another wonderful addition to your accessory wardrobe as a new mother will be pretty hair clips and ponytail holders. That does not mean the boring black ouch-less elastics. It means fashion forward clips and elastics with embellishments, flowers, feathers, and bling. These trendy little bands and clips can quickly and easily take you from baby play date to the grocery store, and back again.

Keep a stash of these at the ready because you will never know when you will need to perk up your look to get you ready for an impromptu outing.

How to Build an Outfit around a Chic Accessory

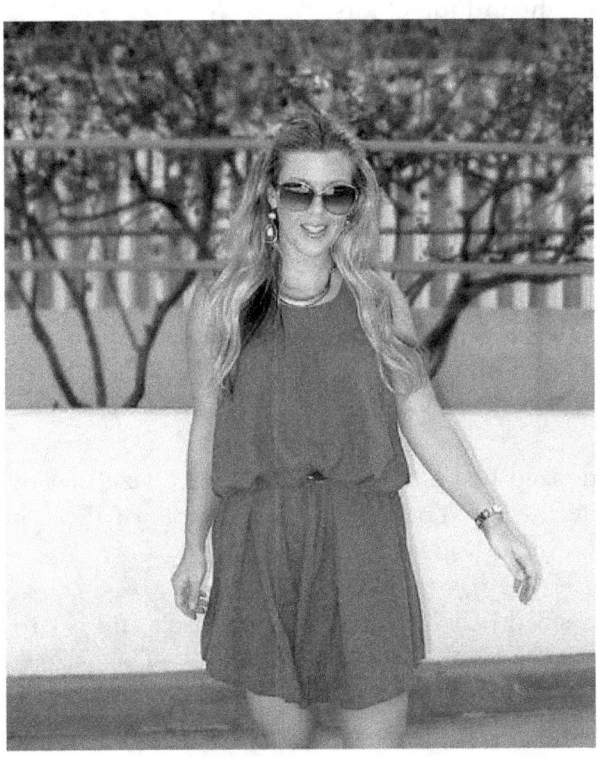

Accessories are the icing on the cake of your stylish and chic outfit. Sure, it would be just as good without them, but think of how much more complete the cake looks with icing! When you are planning accessory additions to your stylish and chic wardrobe, remember to include something from each of the following categories: Belts, shoes, scarves, jewellery, bags, hats, and sunglasses.

Once upon a time, belts were thought of as a strictly utilitarian wardrobe staple. You needed them to hold your pants up. Today; however, they are so much more than that support piece that keeps your Calvin's covered. Today, belts opened a whole new world of stylish embellishment.

Belts come in many different materials, colors, and styles, and are available in three main sizes: Skinny, Medium, and wide. Trends right now find belts being sought after in metallic finishes, leather, braided materials, and embellished with studs. Of course, plain belts are also available in bright and fun colors.

Belts that are approximately one inch wide are classified as skinny belts. These belts are not usually used for holding things up; they are generally used as an accent piece that highlights your waist in your outfit. For example, these are often paired with fun floral rompers done up loosely around the waist in a bright white or other neon color to highlight your waistline.

Skinny belts are more of a minimalist style and are often seen coupled with slim fitting clothing. Large bulky pieces would be lost with these skinny belts.

The medium sized belt is the more traditional size that most of us are already familiar with. You may have a couple of these in your closet already!

The medium sized belt is a very utilitarian belt and is often associated with a very tailored and formalized look. This size belt fits very comfortably in the belt loops of your average pants and helps create a very polished look when worn with a tucked in tailored shirt.

You can find a lot of very fun and fashionable styles of medium sized belts. Braided is a style that has come back on to the radar as well as belts that are studded in a metallic finish. These belts can add some fun to your otherwise formal look by offering a brief peek of your personality and fashion flare.

Wide belts are very on trend right now, and have been for a few seasons. These belts are usually elasticized and offer an oversized fun buckle. These belts are not going to be much help holding up your pants. They are for a fashion look only. Their main purpose is to cinch your waist and draw attention there. These wide belts are often worn slightly higher than a traditional belt and can offer an "empire waistline" view.

These belts can also be very handy in layering styles. Their oversized looks can balance out the bulky sweaters and other more flowing styles, like the swing cardigan.

These belts are readily available in neutrals like black, white and beige, as well as in fun and funky patterns that will really showcase your style and flare in a fun way.

Footwear should always be a consideration when dressing! Your footwear can affect the overall appearance of your outfit. Imagine if one of Hollywood's greatest starlets stepped out on the red carpet wearing a beautiful designer dress that elicited "oohs" and "aahs" from the paparazzi only to reveal a brightly colored rubber clog when she stepped away. The footwear message does not match that of the rest of the outfit! Make sure that your feet are speaking the same language as the rest of your outfit.

Footwear trends often border on the artistic and focus less on the practical. Not many people can spend a day in six inch heels and still have happy feet and non-broken ankles by the end of the day. On the other hand, if you can wear them, more power to you! The greater challenge with footwear is to find a marriage of comfort and style that will keep you and your feet happy all day long!

For those comfort loving fashion fans out there, the wedge is still comfortably in style this season! You will find them in a variety of styles, prints, and materials, not to mention a variety of heel heights. The wedge will offer you more stability in a heel and normally provides more coverage for your foot which translates into more support.

The kitten heel, (a very short ½ - 1" heel) is also refreshingly back in style this season. These heels are low and stable and offer a lot of versatility to move from professional events to fun social events without much effort.

Sky high heels are always there on the fashion foreground for the very confident and well-balanced individuals. Platform heels have also re-surfaced this year and are making a great impact on the traditional sky high. Sky highs or stilettos will often offer you a heel of no less than 3 ½ - 4".

Gladiator sandals are still big this year with a slight variation from last year. This year's sandals offer a more Grecian inspiration than battle forward gladiators. They are softer and more feminine, offering multiple ankle ties and rings in refreshing metallic.

Booties are still making a huge presence this season. The summer ankle bootie with toe cut outs and interesting embellishments certainly are bringing variety to the orthodox Capri partners.

This season shoes are showing up in a variety of micro-suede's in a multitude of colors. Cobalt blue, electric pink and chocolate browns are making a huge impact in all styles. The animal print trend is also translating into footwear with many shoes. Pumps are showing up in leopard print and sky high heels with zebra stripes: either would elevate last season's little black dress to this season's show stopper!

Scarves are another really fantastic way to update your fashionable wardrobe. They offer an opportunity to bring texture and color to some of your otherwise less impact pieces.

Blue jeans and t-shirts can immediately be elevated from casual classification to high fashion when you add a scarf with an interesting and on trend color or print.

Wearing a scarf can be less impact if you are not sure of what to do with it. There are many ways to wear a fashion scarf: You can knot them as you would have winter scarf: loop them around your neck so that the tails hang in the front; fold them in half, loop them around your neck and pull the tail through the loop; wear them as a shawl or in your hair; and your options are endless.

What is a chic and stylish outfit with statement jewellery? Statement jewellery is considered any piece of jewellery that really brings a wow factor to your outfit. This may not help you determine what that is, but suffice to say that you will know it when you see it. Oftentimes, it is the one piece of jewellery that you just cannot take your eyes off of.

Earrings are always a great way to add a hint of your fashion sense and to personalize your outfit. This season feathers are really big and earrings adorned with feathers are all the rage.

Sizes and colors of earrings are definitely a consideration when looking at the stylish and chic wardrobes of the day. If it is a statement piece that does not necessarily mean that it has to be over the top and huge, but it also doesn't mean that it won't be!

If you are selecting some fun and fashionable hoop earrings for example, in a cool neon hue, try to keep them to a reasonable size so as to not channel the throw back to the 1980s vibe that huge hoops would bring.

Sometimes a statement earring can be a beautifully crafted pair of diamond studs which are always fashionable and chic, or sometimes they can be prismatic dangling orbs which are very stylish right now. Remember the vibe that you want to send out, and choose your statement pieces accordingly.

This season when you are looking at rings, cocktail rings are still very popular and the bigger the better. Floral motifs are springing up everywhere as are colored "diamonds" or cubic zirconium. Animal patterns are showing up on thick cocktail rings also, with some very memorable ones showing up with black and white crystals in a zebra stripe pattern.

Costume jewellery is still very popular and offers a lot of great looks that will compliment your stylish ensemble. Colors, styles, and sizes vary greatly which will guarantee that you can find something that will work for you!

Necklaces run the trend path as well as other fashions do. Pearls are back in style, if they ever went out, and are showing up in great big gumball sizes as well as in a variety of different colors. Long strands of pearls are also still very popular, but bring in more subtle pastel hues.

Watches are functional items that you can use to your advantage to quickly and effortlessly update your wardrobe to reflect some of the newest and most stylish trends. This season the "jelly" band watch is very popular especially in very vibrant colors like pure white, lemon yellow, and deep purple.

The size of your watch face can update your wardrobe greatly. Small, delicate watch faces are always on the radar and offer a very chic feel, but the trendiest watches for women are showing up in oversized faces that are embellished with crystals and different colors.

Purses, clutches, and wallets are another quick and easy way to update your style. Today, the style of the bag is more focused on than the material used to create it. On the runway and in stores today you can find hobo bags, totes, shoulder bags, clutches, cross body bags, satchels and almost any other style you can imagine in a variety of prints and colors.

Polka dots and animal prints in bright colors are very trendy right now on bags and can instantly update your look. By adding a hot pink polka dot shoulder bag to your wardrobe, you can immediately modernize your standard black leather jacket.

Remain trendy to the core by making sure that your wallet matches or at least compliments your bag. A more neutral wallet can work with multiple bag options and can keep your entire look streamlined.

Hats are especially big in the summer months and they offer a fun and functional way to keep the sun off your head. If you remember the episode of the television show "Friends" when Rachel wore her gigantic hat to the group's beach house retreat, you will remember her sharing with her group that "hats are back in". They are back in again, although not quite in such a "big" way!

Soft, feminine hats are back this season in fun and flirty colors with boldly colored floral embellishments that may take you back to your childhood. Floppy hats made of natural material like raffia are showing up on the most stylish and trendy beaches, farmers markets, and outdoor concerts. So ditch that trusty old bucket "Gilligan" style hat and find a fashion forward bonnet that will keep those harmful rays off your beautiful face and show the world that you are a fashion force to be reckoned with.

Sometimes it is funny to really look at how fashion influences our health. Sunglasses have been very big style points over the last few years which seem to show how the fashion industry is identifying their usefulness as well as their beauty.

Aviator glasses have been in and out of style since Tom Cruise first sported them in "Top Gun" back in 1986, and they are back in style today! The classic aviator style includes a dark tint on a slightly oval lens that is framed in metal.

Oversized sunglasses with lenses and frames that cover a large part of your cheekbones and above your eyebrows have been in style for a few seasons and offer a great variety of frame choices: tortoise shell is a popular one, but neon hues and standard black with embellishments are also strong choices.

While the aviator and oversized glasses are still on the fashion radar this season, the truly chic and stylish woman is being seen sporting cats' eye framed sunglasses. The cats' eye style, which has been no doubt popularized by Hollywood's nostalgic trip through the 1960s of late, is a sideways oval frame that comes to a point as it approaches the ear. This style is often seen in the classic tortoise shell, but is also very fashionable and impact in animal prints like zebra and tiger stripes, as well as in strong colors like purple and blue.

When you are looking at accessories, do not minimize the importance of other items like bracelets (thick cuff styles and skinny stacking bracelets are both very popular right now), patterned nylons and tights (color is huge! Neon tights with a black shift dress was a fashion favorite of the season previews), and cell phone covers (using your cell phone case to send a message with pre-printed or design your own cover styles are both very on trend right now!). When assembling your fashion face, everything you wear or take with you has a voice. What are you really saying?

Chapter 4: The Stylish Accessories

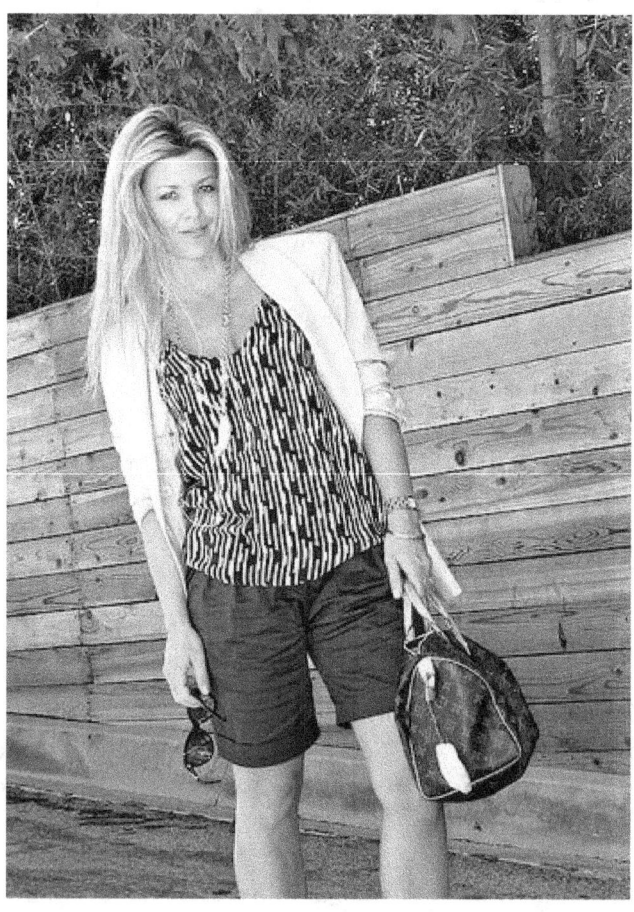

How to Accessorize Chic and Stylish

When you are looking at your closet and deciding how to accessorize your outfit, go with pieces that you love and that work together, but do not feel that you have to wear all of your favorite pieces at once. In fact, doing so can make it look like you're trying too hard.

The most stylish and chic women know that one key piece is enough when they are dressing on trend. A well-chosen accessory can be very impactful when it is played up properly. For example, pair a solid bold colored accessory with a fun printed tunic to play up the color match, and leave it at that!

If your top is embellished, then think about ditching the necklace in favor of a bold statement bracelet or pair of shoes. Do not overwhelm your outfit with too much bling and glitz. Doing so will quickly move your status from a fashion template to a fashion failure.

Wearing one on trend piece at a time is also a very good idea. Adding animal prints in hot metallic colors with neon undertones will just start to make you look like a clown. Know when to say when. Wear one key piece at a time, and be remembered for the chic and stylish way you put together that outfit, as opposed to being remembered for the trail of glitter and giggles you left behind.

Color is an important element to think about when you are dressing on trend. For example, you can include multiple accessories in an outfit as long as they complement each other and don't compete for your attention.

A black sleeveless shift dress worn with a skinny black patent leather belt, black micro-suede wedges would be very impactful with a statement bracelet like a thick zebra striped cuff bracelet or interestingly pattered scarf; but not with both.

How to Get Stylish Accessories

Accessories are everywhere, and all it takes is a little imagination and an open mind.

There is very little you can do to personalize clothing items, and they are a big part of your ensemble, so they are very noticeable.

When it comes to accessories, however, you have a bit more flexibility because you can add personal touches to them to make them truly yours, and you can wear them differently than everyone else!

To find the hottest accessories, shop around. They can turn up in the most unlikely places. Sometimes the accessory shops (the stores dedicated to stocking only fashionable accessories like "Claires" and "Ardenes") can be great places to find on trend items that you can make your own. Often their prices are very reasonable and there is enough of a selection that you won't be guaranteed to be wearing the same watch as every other woman on the bus.

Chain stores that focus on one accessory, like shoes, can be a great place to find fashionable and stylish items. While stores like "Payless Shoe Source" had a questionable fashion name in their early years be assured that they would not still be around if they were not providing a fashionable and accessible option to their customers.

Other times, department stores may be your best bet. They can often bring them to the market very quickly and offer some interesting interpretations of the hottest styles. They can also be the first place that everyone else goes to and with their buyers purchasing mass quantities of the same item may make the items less individualized.

Lower end stores may surprise you by bringing in some of the biggest fashion trends quite quickly and at a very reasonable price. These stores may not be the first stop for the average fashionista which means that the items you find there may be uniquely yours.

Smaller retailers may also be a great resource for finding chic and stylish accessories. They often have a much more personal relationship with their suppliers and can get their hands on very interesting and unique items that will be sure to find a place in your "statement gallery". Having a small retailer on your side can prove to be quite beneficial when you are looking for key trendy pieces. Nurturing these relationships can really pay off in the end.

Thrift and consignment stores can offer you a really interesting perspective on accessories, especially for those trends that have been around before in some manifestation. Vintage finds of new trends can really increase your fashion individualism because you will be assured that not everyone will be sporting the same iconic piece you have.

With accessories, you will be surprised at how many closet fashion designers are out there peddling their wares on the internet. Many of these designers pride themselves on remaining very current with the fashion trends and will use the runway as inspiration for their own styles.

These items can be found quite reasonably priced on the internet and in the end you can feel good knowing that you are contributing to the global economy by supporting an entrepreneur.

When you are looking for chic and stylish accessories, you can also choose to go right to the designer's house to purchase these items. If your budget supports it, then buying accessories directly from the designer will guarantee that you are sporting a one of a kind piece.

How to Make a Stylish Hair Accessory

If you are someone who has an artistic eye and the ability to be creative, then making your own accessories can be a relaxing and rewarding hobby for you.

There are many different sites on the internet that can offer your advice on how to create a stylish hair accessory, but don't rely only on them. Use your creativity to design your own styles that use the fashion trends that are out there right now.

For example, when Prince William and Katherine Middleton got married, there was a huge resurgence of the popularity of the fascinator and they were showing up everywhere on the runway and in stores. Some of the designer labels were selling them for upwards of $200.00.

The cleaver and crafty fashionista was able to reproduce the style with the help of her local craft store for only a few dollars. Stylishly putting together some feathers and some interesting embellishments on a felt base with hot glue then attaching it to a bobby pin or comb saved her quite a bit of money, and allowed her to produce a product that would be truly hers along.

Designing your own jewellery using some of the trends out there is another way to really personalize your style and express your individuality.

What are the Basic Accessories that are Safe yet Stylish for Men?

Sadly, men always seem to get the short end of the fashion stick. There are not a lot of options for them outside the norm.

High end men's fashions offer more options, but are often not accessible to the average man. There are, however, three key pieces that every man should have in his repertoire to keep him looking fashionable and on trend.

Belts, while not as fun and variable as women's belts, can still help a man show his fashion knowledge. Men's belts are generally found in one standard width and in either black or brown. Their buckles, however, can really give you a sense of their fashion sense.

Of course there are the large oversized belt buckles that may show a flag, team logo, or other popular culture reference. These are certainly expressive and show the man's individuality; however, they are not considered very stylish.

A stylish belt buckle will speak more about the material, size and shape of the buckle. A very trendy buckle right now is squared off, medium sized, and is a brushed metal, usually pewter or gun metal.

Rounded buckles with braided leather belts are very reminiscent of the 1980s Miami Vice craze and will not paint you in a very trendy light. And very few men can pull off a white or neon skinny belt, so it is best to remain conservative in your fashion choices and stick with the neutral colors.

Watches are another great place for men to show their fashion savvy. A wide dialled face with a dark background and interesting features show that a man is up on his fashion details. Wearing a brightly colored Swatch Watch ® of the 1980s or anything with a Velcro strap or digital face will not give that same impression.

Jack Nicholson knows how important sunglasses are to the average man. He once told a fashion magazine reporter "What my sunglasses on, I am Jack Nicholson. Without them I am fat and 60".

Sunglasses are a great way for a man to personalize his brand. Aviator styles are chic and sexy and work for almost every face shape. The mirrored or dark tint lens offers an element of mystery, which is also very chic and stylish.

Sports inspired sunglasses, which are favored by many men, are great to use on the sports field. For a night out on the town or other events that don't involve team activities; however, he should have a more stylish pair at the ready that will complete the stylish and trendy package he is creating.

Must Have Basic Accessories

As has already been discussed, accessories can add just the right finishing touch to the fashionable ensemble you are creating. While there are hundreds of options out there for accessories you can choose, focus your attention on the following items to ensure that your outfits will make the grade.

Sunglasses are huge because you wear them front and center on your face, they can very quickly demonstrate how fashion forward you are, or just as quickly date you. You can swiftly alter your fashion tone by investing in a new pair of sunglasses that reflect the hottest trends. Right now, the hottest sunglasses are being snatched up in neon and animal print patterns on a cat's eye style frame.

Another really quick way to update your style is to commit to upgrading your bag to match the trends of the season. The bag you choose will show the world where you stand on the fashion front, so make sure it shouts out loud and clear that you have your finger on the pulse of fashion. The coolest bags this season are showing up as slings and pouches in vibrant neon colors.

Similarly, updating your purse with a one trend style will showcase your fashion savvy to the world. The styles that take first prize this season include really cool and interesting clutches in unnatural animal prints.

Jewellery generally falls into two categories: Timeless and trendy. Timeless jewellery is always in style and always looks chic and stylish. Some examples of timeless jewellery are sleeper hoops, simple gold chains, and classic stud earrings. These pieces are generally something that you invest money in and plan to keep for a long time.

Trendy jewellery on the other hand is usually more accessible and will only be kept in the foreground of your wardrobe for a season or two. Updating your jewellery with a key trendy piece each season is a great way to keep your style fresh. Animal prints, natural elements, and gold are all very hot this season, so incorporate them if you can.

A no-brainer way to immediately update your wardrobe is by adding in a hot and trendy footwear style. This season, menswear inspiration is everywhere including footwear. Lace up oxfords in cool colors will instantly bring your wardrobe up-to-date.

Sandals and boots are also great ways to bring your fashionable footwear to the foreground of your wardrobe. Choose pieces that will compliment your current wardrobe and will help your transition through the seasons in comfort and style.

Make up is another accessory that you shouldn't neglect. Following fashion trends with your make up can quickly take your face to a new fashionable level.

Lately the retro styles of old Hollywood have been dominating the red carpet. This means very often that you select to play up one of your two main features; either your eyes or your lips. Soft and feminine eye makeup in peaches and neutrals is often complimented with a strong red lip. The smoky eye fashion can also be a very striking feature provided it coupled with a soft lip.

Be sure to keep the makeup balanced out because otherwise it will be competing against itself and you will look terribly overdone and not nearly as stylish or chic as you hope to.

If you are wearing a key statement piece, then keep your make up soft and subtle. Too many focal points will only overwhelm you in your attempt to be chic and stylish.

Chapter 5: Your Crowning Glory

What Kinds of Hairstyles are Professional, Chic and Feminine?

Your hair is the ultimate accessory when you are a chic and stylish woman! Everything from the cut to the color to the style speaks volumes about you.

When you are visualizing a high powered professional woman, many things should jump out at you: the way she enters a room, the clothes she wears, and her hair. It is hard to be taken seriously in a ponytail or Dorothy Hamill hair cut; it doesn't mean that you need to wear a hard solemn hair style, either, though.

It does mean that you need to update your hair style regularly. Hair is a tricky subject because it is such a part of our identity and we are often resistant to change. However, if you look back at pictures from five years ago and your hair style hasn't changed, then there is no way that you are projecting the stylish and chic image that you could be.

When deciding on a style, start by determining your face shape. An oval face is longer than it is round; a square face shape is just that; a heart shaped face is broader at the forehead and pointier at the chin; a triangular face shape has a wider chin with less pronounced forehead; a diamond shaped face has a pointed chin and narrow forehead; round faces are approximately as wide as they are long; and oblong faces generally look like a softer rectangle.

Each face shape lends itself to a more successful style. You cannot change the shape of your face (without extensive plastic surgery), so it is a much better idea to work within it.

There are many sites online that will offer you suggestions on the type of haircut and style that will work with your face shape, and that is a great place to start, but there are other factors to consider when looking at the hot trends.

For example, not everyone has a face like Halle Berry, so her super short pixie hair cut that was all the rage in the mid-2000s was not a style that everyone should have embraced.

The texture of your hair is another factor that will affect which styles you can employ. A piecey, texturized cut that looks good on a woman with naturally curly hair will fall short on someone with poker straight hair, no matter what products she employs.

Color trends come and go, too, and your skin tone can dramatically alter how a color that looks amazing on one woman looks on you. Not everyone can rock the platinum blonde trend that is out there right now, but almost everyone can find a variation of the color trend that will work on them.

Picking a style that is professional, chic, and feminine can be a difficult task to undertake alone, so enlist the help of professionals. Pay for a consultation with a professional hair stylist if you have to. Sometimes the pain of paying your hard-earned money to hear "no" is worth not having to live with a terrible fashion faux pas!

Today's hottest styles include long flowing, messy beach waves; simple bangs; and interesting elements (like side braids). The colors seen most often on the runway this year is a platinum blonde and dark auburn; although a multitude of rainbow colors have also been seen.

Remember that the exact style and color that is hot and trendy on one person may not work for you. Develop a relationship with your hair stylist and be sure that you can trust them. A respectful relationship will allow your stylist to be frank and honest with you when you come in with an unrealistic expectation.

If you are working with a consummate "yes man" in your hairstylist then you need to think about moving on. You undoubtedly spend good money on your hair style and you deserve to get a style that looks professional and chic on you. If your stylist cannot say no to you, you may find yourself stuck with something that looks more like a poodle cut than the mod bob you were hoping for.

The stylist you work with will also have a really good idea of how to work with your hair to achieve the style you are looking for. If it is a possibility, then knowing your hair will allow your stylist to be successful.

Hair color can also keep you looking on trend. If you are open to changing your current color, or just kicking it up a notch, then consider moving towards the blonde or auburn family by consulting with a professional who will help you select the appropriate hues to compliment your skin tone.

When you choose to chemically change your hair color, you are committing to keeping it up. There is nothing stylish or chic about letting your roots or grey hair show through. Work with your stylist to find a color that may not require as much extensive upkeep. If you choose to jump on board the color bandwagons for this season, be aware that both blondes and reds require quite a bit of upkeep to maintain the "fresh from the salon" look and feel.

Regardless of the style you choose, a chic, professional, and feminine hair style is always clean, polished, and out of your face. Hiding behind rogue bangs all day makes you look more like a self-conscious teenager than the strong and confident woman that you are.

If you do happen to embark on a very wrong style path, find that great hat you picked out and keep those stylish hair accessories at the ready.

It is not the end of the world. Remember, the difference between a good hair style and a bad hair style is about four weeks!

What Kind of Hairstyle is Suitable for Students in High school?

Adolescence is a time for experimentation with fashion and that includes hair. Hair colors, cuts and styles are always changing in a typical high school classroom.

There are always a variety of styles seen in high school from ultra long hair to super short; natural hair colors, to cotton candy pink. Some styles are very on trend and some are very classics.

Today's hottest teen hair styles come from the punk world. The essence of a punk hairstyle is its weirdness and color. Some traditional punk styles have included Mohawks and rainbow colors, but today, the punk looks much softer and more accessible.

The punk styling of today's teens really brings out their inner confidence and because of the wide variety of styles that fall under this umbrella, it does tend to compliment most face shapes.

Punk styling can include choppy layers of varying lengths, asymmetrical styling, long sweeping bangs, and a huge array of colors. Shaved designs, spiked bangs, and over the top artistic colors are other characteristics that are common in punk hair.

The singers P!nk and Avril Lavinge both had a hand in bringing the punk style to a mainstream audience and are considered the founding mothers of the style. They popularized what was traditionally a "rebellious" style and make it more accessible and acceptable to the masses.

The non-punk trend shows long side swept bangs with classic or edgier styling.

Clean, polished, and tidy hair will always make your style more fashionable and chic. Experiment and have fun with your hair.

What are Some Cute Hair Styles for a Scene/ Emo Chic?

According to Wikipedia, emo is a style of rock music influenced fashion that is characterized by wearing slim fit pants and rock t-shirts. They characterize the hair styles as including side swept bangs which may cover one or both eyes, super straight hair with choppy layers that are either bleached blonde or dyed jet black with highlights of red, pink, blue or other bright colors.

How to Look Polished and Stylish with Very Long or Very Short Hair

The basis of a good hair style that will keep you looking polished and stylish is to start with a good cut. Work with a stylist you trust and be very clear with your communication.

Be wary of very long hair. If it is left at one length it can very quickly weigh you down and make you look much older than your years. While many women really like to wear their hair super long and one length it is very hard to keep it looking trendy.

Length is something that you can work with in a hair style as long as you are flexible enough to work with some layering. Your hair will look much fresher and more stylish if it is able to move independently in its layers.

For both short and long hair, regular maintenance is important in keeping it looking polished and stylish. Keeping the split ends trimmed and sustain the shape of the cut during growth are two things you can do very easily that can really help keep you looking good.

Use hair accessories to keep your style fresh and trendy. Embellished bobby pins, hair clips, and head bands can really help keep your hair fashionable, regardless of the length.

Get to know your products. Treat your hair right and keep it healthy. Use the appropriate products for your style and for what you want to get out of it. Smoothers will help to tame the fly aways that you may have and will give you a sleek looks. Pomades can help to texturize your hair and twist it into the shape and style you are looking for. Leave in conditioners may be a great choice for your hair provided you find one that works with your hair's chemistry and doesn't leave it looking beaten down and oily.

Tips on How to Get Chic and Stylish Bangs

Bangs are a huge commitment when you are looking at a hair trend. Bangs can help to frame your face and emphasis your eyes. They can be dramatic with a straight shortcut or soft with an angled blended cut.

Bang styles today are leaning away from the harsh dramatic bangs of the early 1990s and are focusing more on the softer, more flowing feminine bangs.

Regardless of the style of bangs you embrace, do yourself a favor and consult a professional! This is not the time for you to break out your scissors and complete a do it yourself project.

As mentioned before, a good hair stylist will be able to tell you if your hair is suitable to be cut into bangs. A very curly hair style may not be a good choice for bangs unless you are committed to drying and straightening them every morning.

It takes a very long time for hair to grow out, at the snails pace of 0.5 inches a month, so be sure that you know what you (or whoever is cutting your hair) knows what they are doing!

What is the Most Stylish Hair Cut for Your Face?

Every haircut is an individual choice. What looks great on your best friend may not work on you at all. It is so very important to remember that when you are looking at pictures of hairstyles.

Not everyone is meant to have the same style. Do you remember the "Rachel Green" layered shag hair cut that came from the television show "Friends"? It was reportedly the most requested haircut ever at the time, and there were literally thousands of women walking the street with a haircut that really didn't work for them at all!

Think about your lifestyle when you're choosing a haircut. Stylish haircuts can only be as stylish as you make them. If you are a wash and wear hairstyle person and you choose a haircut that requires blow drying, straightening, and applying product every day you may not be able to stick with the routine for very long, so be honest with yourself about your commitment.

Do not fight nature when you are contemplating a hair style. If you are looking at a picture of Rhianna and are requesting that exact hair style, be prepared for the outcome to not look exactly the same because you are not the person in the picture. You will get a version of that hair style that works on you, with your hair.

How can You Choose an Easy and Stylish Hair Cut?

The best way to go about selecting a hair style that is both on trend and will work for you is to work with a professional.

You will need to do some work on your own before you get to the consultation stage, so start by looking at pictures. Identify what it is that you like about a certain haircut. Do you like the way it hangs, or the structure of it? Is it the color you aspire to have or the length that you like? Knowing what you like will give you a great launching point for a detailed and in-depth conversation with your stylist.

When you are surrounding yourself with pictures and ideas of the style you want to achieve, it is really helpful if you can look at the pictures and ideas as "inspiration" only meaning that there are pieces you like about them and want to aim for, but know that you are not the same person in the picture, so it stands to reason that the hair style will not look the same on you.

Chapter 6: Styling Feet

How to Look Stylish while Wearing Comfortable Shoes

Footwear serves two very different purposes. It is a fun and cute way to update your fashion wardrobe by anchoring your style and it is also a utilitarian piece of clothing that helps you get through the day in comfort. When you are really lucky, you are able to find shoes that accomplish both tasks at the same time!

When you think of comfortable shoes, very often your mind falls back on to a couple of key pieces of footwear: your favorite running shoes; plastic clogs; fuzzy slippers; and fur lined boots. There is no arguing the fact that these are very comfortable; however their style score is almost nothing!

Think about what you like best about these favorite comfortable footwear pieces and try to find those attributes in your stylish and chic ones! For example, if you find out that you really do like the low heel, or flats, and it is important to you that they have a generous cut in the toes so your feet don't get all cramped, then you will have an excellent place to start when you are shoe shopping.

If that is the case, then stay away from anything over a 2" heel and look for shoes with a charitable cut in the toes. You can still embrace the pointy toed styles that are out there today, you just may need to try on a slightly larger size to allow your toe's room to move!

Sometimes when you find the perfect pair of shoes to compliment your outfit, or you just find a pair that you have fallen in love with, the fit isn't exactly what you are looking for. If it is a sizing problem, such as the shoe, is too narrow or small for your foot then there really isn't much opportunity for you to play with that. Find the right size or you will have problems later!

If however, the shoe is too large, you can purchase inserts that will help to re-size your shoes and make them the appropriate size for your foot.

Many times when you are looking at women's dress shoes, the insert of the shoe doesn't appear to offer you much support. And there is nothing more uncomfortable than walking on the sidewalk and being able to feel every pebble underfoot.

Check out your local footwear department or pharmacy and investigate the gel and cushion inserts you can purchase for your footwear. Adding a gel inserts or even a pillow cushion pad can really adjust the feel of your shoes and can take them from a one-time wear to a new favorite. Just remember that adding this insert can require you to adjust the size of the shoe. You really do not have to sacrifice comfort for style!

Tips on Stylish Shoes for Casual Wearing

Casual shoes are often relegated to "casual" status for good reason. Sometimes they are a favorite pair of 10 year old sneakers, and sometimes they are those wonderfully comfortable plastic clogs. No matter what they are, if they are ugly or in poor repair, then they are not helping you put your best fashion foot forward.

Shoes that you wear with casual outfits do not have to be ugly to be comfortable. There are some really cute and stylish choices out there this year and with the right guidance and mindset you can find the casual shoe that will carry you through all of your casual gatherings this season.

In the summer, it is easy to fall into the plastic flip flop trap and slide them on with everything you wear. They are comfortable and do come in a variety of fashion colors, but they are not the best choice when putting together a stylish and chic outfit.

Flip flops do have their place in your current wardrobe, and that should be in the bathroom or at the beach or poolside. They are very fun and functional footwear, but not stylish in the least.

If you are a flip flop lover, then take a look in the shoe department the next time you are out and you will be amazed at the beautiful, stylish, and trendy sandals you can find out there that really echo the flip flop feel without the flip flop fashion fail.

Many sandals this summer are showing a flip flop influence with the leather foot bed, embellished toe thong and kitten heel or wedge. This slight variation on the flip flop elevates the otherwise too casual shoe into something that can take you from work to the weekend in style.

Other sandal styles this season can really bring you out of your flip flop rut. Strappy is still key this season and it seems that the more straps the better. Look for strappy sandals with or without an ankle strap and with varying heights of heels.

Color and prints abound on this season's footwear from sandals to pump, so choose one that will flatter your wardrobe and keep you looking fresh all season long.

Some individuals are married to their sneakers or running shoes. Your brand name footwear cradles your foot, offers you support, and just generally makes your foot look good. While there are plenty of interesting color combinations and styles out there, no matter what you do to them, they still look like they belong in the gym.

Running shoes with your shorts is not a fashion forward image. But if you cannot break yourself of the sneaker trend, then look for a stylish option that will give you the same feel, but with a trendier outcome.

There are many options out there that will offer you the same sporty feel of your sneakers with a more stylish face. For, example a pair of plain leather sneakers with minimal logos and grommets can help your transition from your gym rat look to a more sophisticated fashionista.

The praises of the ballet flat have already been sung, but they warrant another chorus. Ballet flats, which are available in a variety of colors and patterns offer you great versatility and can look equally in place with a casual wrap dress as they can with jeans or Capri's.

The embellishments on your ballet flats are another way to tell from which season they come. Last year's simple and sweet ribbon styling on the toe has been replaced by this season's bling and pizzazz.

Micro suede, fuzzy animal print, and patent finishes are all equally beautiful in ballet flats and can really raise the level of your standard black bottoms.

Nautical inspired foot wear is also a big trend this year. The stylish and chic woman has at least one pair of "boat shoes" in her closet. These preppy loafer style shoes are easy to slip on and come in a variety of feminine and fun colors. The added bonus with these shoes is that they were built for stability and comfort. You will not find any super high heels attached here, and the insides of the shoes are almost slipper like.

No matter what the season boots can always help you transition your style. This season the bootie sandal is being seen everywhere: with varying heel heights, details, and colors, the peep toe summer bootie is for the most confident and fashion forward dressers.

In the spring and fall season previews this year, booties have been seen everywhere as has the standard equestrian riding boot. Booties offer an easy dressing choice and can be found in a variety of styles, colors and patterns.

Equestrian styling has been big for the last few seasons and continues to make a presence this season with the mid-calf height boots. Lacing details and the comfortable flat heel make these boots a welcome addition to everyone woman's wardrobe.

The continuing trend of the skinny pant makes the bootie and boot choice an easy one. They can really polish off what could be a thrown together outfit and give it a very polished and classy look.

Styling Up a Cheap Pair of Shoes to Look Unique and Chic

Cheap does not mean ugly. There are many companies out there that sell "throw away" footwear which means that it is uber trendy right now and won't live out the season, so you can purchase the style quite reasonably. Pay-less Shoe Source is one of the best known companies right now. They offer a variety of styles for men women and children at very reasonable price points to allow everyone the opportunity to be on trend with their footwear.

There are many "one season" options out there for your footwear choices at many different price points. The challenge with shopping at well priced retailers for current on trend fashion items is that just about everyone else in your community is probably shopping there too, so odds are you will end up seeing your shoes on someone else.

You can work with many easy items to personalize your more economically priced footwear to make it uniquely your own.

If you are crafty or have an artistic inspiration, you can very easily add embellishments to your footwear that will make them stand out as yours alone. The biggest challenge is to keep them looking chic and stylish and not turn them into a telltale art project.

Black ballet flats can quickly and easily be updated by adding on a store bought hair clip in a hot fashion trend. For example, adding an alligator clip with a sparkly black and white peony to each shoe can really bring last year's style to the forefront.

If you are more daring you can add a glitter spray to your old outdated flats or heels to instantly increase their bling appeal and add some drama to their tired silhouette.

Iron on or seem and stick fabric decals can be an interesting option to add to your footwear to keep them on trend and stylish. Adding a bit of bling in a floral print or animal inspiration can keep you very fashion forward.

The biggest and best way to personalize your inexpensive footwear to make them look stylish and chic is to wear them with the proper attitude. Fashion has a lot to do with the clothes that you wear, but it also has more to do with HOW you wear them. If you love them, wear them with pride and confidence, no matter what you spent on them!

Stylish and Comfortable Alternatives to Pumps

When it comes to footwear, your options are almost unlimited. There are many different comfortable and stylish options out there that can replace your tired and back straining pumps.

Flats are always an option when reworking your fashion footwear. They are low to the ground, built for comfort, and always make your outfit look polished.

Some women want to include the additional height of heels, so in those cases, flats are not an option for them. When you want to add some height to your frame with fashion footwear, but want to avoid wearing pumps then think about wedges: the heel lover's best friend.

Wedges offer a slightly higher than standard heel (at approximately 3" although they are available in other heights, too), with a more stable, thicker sole. Having a solid sole allows your shoe to have more contact with the ground which not only allows you to be more stable when walking, but also allows your body weight to be spread out over the entirety of the sole: Thus eliminating the shock points of walking on a 1" square heel.

Wedges seem to have remained on the fashion radar for the last few years, even with the fluctuation of heel sizes. No matter what the key on trend piece is, the classic and comfortable wedge can fit the bill with the appropriate material, color, or pattern.

Choosing the Right Shoes for your Outfit

There are times when you buy a pair of shoes and build your outfit around them, and then there are times when you have the outfit and have to match them to your shoes. When you are matching shoes to your outfit, you need to take a holistic approach to the outfit and ensure that they absolutely go together.

Look at the tone of your outfit. Are you putting together a fun and breezy outfit with flowing material and soft colors? If you are, then dark chunky shoes would cut off your outfit with a visual break. You would want to make sure that your footwear echo's the feeling of your outfit and keep them light and airy looking as well.

When dressing, you will need to keep the purpose of the event in mind. If it is a formal occasion, then you are best to opt for something dressy and heels are the natural fit. Remember that sneakers are for the gym, and flip flops are for the beach.

Keep in mind what you will need to do in that outfit! If you are going to be on your feet for an extended period of time, then you may wish to rethink your sky high heels and opt for something that is lower and will offer you more stability and comfort for the day. Kitten heels, wedges, and flats can all be very fashionable and trendy and offer you more staying power than those 6" heels. There is nothing more frustrating than being at a social event and wanting to stay out on the floor dancing or mingling, but your aching feet have relegated you to sitting on the sideline.

Colors can be tricky when matching shoes to outfits. You will most likely never match the colors perfectly, so do not even try! A slightly mismatched coloring can really take away from your otherwise beautiful outfit. When dealing in bold colors, work with contrast and make it obvious that you weren't trying to match it up perfectly. Pick a bold color from your stylishly patterned outfit and highlight it with your footwear.

Too much matching can make you look more like a color by numbers picture than a stylish and chic fashionista. Never underestimate the power of a metallic shoe when you are dressing for fashion. Silvers, golds, pewters, and bronzes can be very accommodating with your fashion choices and can add an element of sophistication that you just cannot match with a matched up color choice.

A good rule of thumb when matching your shoes to your outfit is to remember to compliment your clothing rather than your outfit. What that means simply is that patterned shoes go really well with simple outfits. If your outfit is looking a bit bland then add in those fun patterned shoes and kick your outfit up a notch.

It seems simple and like it doesn't even need to be said, but make sure that your footwear is season appropriate for the outfit. If you are looking at a New Year's Eve outfit and have a wonderful party dress, don't make it look uneven by strapping on your summer sandals. Instead, weigh it out evenly with dark tights and cute fashion booties that will allow you to stay warm and dance the night away!

Finally, evaluate the overall effect. Does it work for you? Do you absolutely love the overall look of the outfit from top to bottom? If you do, then go with it! A true stylish and chic woman knows what she likes and what looks good on her.

These points are just guidelines, so if you put your shoes with your outfit and you absolutely love it, and then go with it. Your confidence and attitude will direct how the outfit really goes together.

Chapter 7: Styling up the Toes

Stylish Nail Designs

Toe nails are finally getting their place of honor with fashionable designs of their own. Not that long ago, it seemed that French manicures were for fingers only, but judging by the increase of French nail pedicures, the trend of a couple of years back is still going strong.

In the summer months when your toes are getting more air time than usual, it is important to make sure that they are giving the same overall impression as your clothing. You can be dressed very stylishly and on trend, but if your nails are chipped, unpainted, or in poor repair, then they are singing a different tune than the rest of you!

Styling the toes can add the bling and glitz that was usually added by toe rings and ankle bracelets; two fashion trends that seem to be taking the back seat this season.

Nail styling is super hot this season and with the ready accessibility of the do it yourself nail styling pens, these fashion plate styles can be achieved at home for a fraction of the cost and with very little training required!

Polka dots are a fantastic nail trend right now. Adding contrasting polka dots to a solid base coat of toe nail polish can put your otherwise overlooked toes to a fashion pedestal.

To achieve this looks, paint your toes in a solid color of your choosing and let them dry. When they are dry, take a contrasting color of regular nail polish and dip a toothpick in the nail polish. It may be helpful to pour a bit of the nail polish on a plate or throw away spoon to ensure that you are only getting a little bit of polish on the pick. Otherwise, you can very easily smudge the dots or turn them into blobs. Allow the dots to dry completely and then add a top coat of clear sealant protector.

Multi colored crackle polish is also another great way to add style to your toe nails. Paint your nails in any combination of colors that you like, allow them to dry completely, and then apply the crackle coat overlay in a contrasting color on them. When the crackle coat dries it will crack and create breaks in the over color which will allow the undercoat to show through.

The nail polish pens and accent colors as well as jewels and crystals can allow you the opportunity to personalize your toe nails with their simple additions.

There are other products on the market right now that are very fashionable and can instantly transform your toe nails into works of art with butterflies, prints, gems and other details. These products are applied like a sticker to a clean and dry nail. They are cut to fit the nail and smoothed on with a rub stick.

Many of the hot on trend patterns today for nails include floral, nature, neon colors, animal prints, polka dots and stripes.

What Color of Nail Polish is Stylish?

Today, there are many different colors trends for nail polish which makes being on trend accessible for everyone: Colors are huge, both pastel and non-pastel; and neon takes center stage.

Bright neon colors are a fun and fresh way to update your nails and stay on trend. They scream summer and offer a carefree feeling of youth. If you are not comfortable with the light colors on your hands, then you can be equally on trend with a soft and muted pastel color. Mauve's and greens are super hot right now and will transition through the seasons very well and you can never go wrong with a bold, solid, on trend color like cobalt blue.

Of course, not everyone is comfortable with a variety of colors on their hands, nor is it appropriate in every workplace. Nicely manicured, well maintained nails with smooth cuticles and clean nails are always stylish and chic and will always lend an air of sophistication to your outfit.

Acrylic Nail Tips

Not everyone is able to grow out their nails due to their body chemistry, nasty habits, or work requirements. And, sometimes you just want to have that elegant, elongated nail on the end of your fingers to finish off your look. You can accomplish this by asking a professional to add acrylic nail tips.

Nail tip styles usually jockey back and forth between the squared off and rounded tips. Today, however, the trend seems to be following Hollywood's fashionistas who prefer the "stiletto" or pointed nail trend. These nails form a point on the tip and visually elongate the fingers.

This style is a very fashionable right now. The functionality of this style depends on your lifestyle. Sporting stiletto style nails while you try to bathe a new born baby, or put in your contact lenses may not work for you.

Like every other fashion trend out there, it is important to evaluate your life style and determine if this one will fit into your life.

Adding Style to Plain Black Nails

A plain black nail can be the most boring paint job ever, or it can open a world of creativity and artistry for you. It all depends on how you see it!

Embellishing your plain black nails can add a new world of style and sex appeal that you never expected. Sometimes something as simple as a sweep of contrasting polish, a strategically placed gem, decal, or polka dot can turn your nails into works of art.

Glitter nail paint can be used to add interesting detail to your nails and with a steady hand and an artist's mind you can instantly create beautiful patterns and images.

Adding words and messages to your nails was a trend popularized by Lindsay Lohan. Using rub on letters or colorful stickers, you can apply them to clean and dry painted nails to spell out the message you want to share. And, sealing it with a clear top coat can preserve the message for days.

Stylish Nails with Art and Polish

There are lots of interesting and fun ways to add stylish components to your finger and toe nails. You are limited only by your imagination.

Start with clean and shaped nails. Then, add a fun and trendy color that you love. Make sure it is something that you can live with for a few days if you are not able to devote the time to it each day. Decide what you want to do with it. Add embellishments that you can buy from the store or freehand in decorations that you love.

Sometimes just a few well-placed strokes of your brush can add in a flower, an interesting dividing line, color blocking, or other really cool options. Experiment with them and find what you like. Search online for inspiring and interesting nail styles and try to copy them yourself, or take them to a professional and see what they can do.

The biggest thing to remember is that your hands are the first things that many people will see when dealing with you. Make sure that they are neat, clean and presentable. Those ten little nails can make a huge impact on your fashionable and chic wardrobe.

Chapter 8: Style on a Budget

How to Buy Stylish Clothing on a Budget

Fashions change every season and keeping up with them can be a very expensive and exhausting job if you don't know where to look.

Fashion bargains are more readily accessible today than they have ever been in fashion history. There was a time when you could only find the newest fashion pieces at the designer's place in another country and they would cost you a small fortune because they were hands sewn and original works.

Today, thanks to the internet and the accessibility of those high end fashion designs for inspiration, many smaller fashion houses are creating their own take on the big designer's collections and offering them to the masses quickly, reasonably, and in their own community.

Being stylish and chic should not be a privilege; it should be your fashionable right, regardless of how much money you have to spend on clothing. Fashion should not break the bank.

Today, most retailers will offer very trendy pieces at quite reasonable prices. In some cases, these trends may be delivered to the public a season or two behind the big designer labels.

Depending on where you live in the world, you may be right on trend with delivery time and you may not. Living in Europe tends to bring people closer to the trends while it seems to take a season or two to cross the ocean and deliver those same styles to North America.

Fortunately, there are some really progressive fashion houses out there who are offering parallel lines of their collections at a high end and more accessible price point. H&M is one of the newest, most fresh fashion retailers in North America right now. They offer very on trend items for men, women, and children that are accessible at the same time they are hitting the runways in Paris.

These fashions are very reasonably priced and offer a good variety of interpretations of the style, which is also a great bonus because maxi dresses do not look good on everyone, nor do micro minis. Options are a great thing in the fashion world.

Familiarize yourself with the big name designers that you love and seek out their outlet opportunities. It may require a bit of a drive, but the savings you can get on stylish items that are hot in the fashion industry may very well make up for the price of gas!

If the name brand itself isn't important to you then keep your eyes open for the style interpretations that you can find. Most department stores carry a version of them at all many different price points. WalMart, for example, has a very fashion forward line of clothing called "George" that offers some very trendy pieces at very low prices.

Develop a good relationship with a small retailer whose items you enjoy. They can often offer a more personal service than a department store can and may even offer to call you when items you like are reduced for the season. The trendy dress at 50% off looks even more attractive!

Consignment stores and thrift stores can be a wealth of great items. Searching through the racks in these stores can be very exciting and finding an Oscar De La Renta cocktail jacket for $10.00 in your size can be a fashionista's dream come true. Finding this season's bags, coats, and shoes can be very easy to do at a fraction of the price making the treasure hunt pay off in droves!

Shopping at consignment and thrift stores will allow you to develop your own identity and can also ensure that you are not showing up at your next social event wearing the same dress as three other party goers.

If you and your friends are all of a-like mind and size then consider hosting a clothes or accessory swap party. Invite your friends to come over with a certain number of accessories or clothing pieces that they don't wear any more or are just ready to rotate through their wardrobes.

Put them out on display around your family room with some wine and cheese, play some fun upbeat tunes, and let everyone shop. Set up a separate room to try on clothing and work out your swap rules. Allow the browsing to start when people arrive, but do not let any of the "shopping" start until the agreed upon time. First come first served; and you all go home with some new and interesting items to work into your existing wardrobe.

How to Make Old Clothes Look New and Stylish

The best way to keep your wardrobe looking fresh season after season is to really analyze the trends and add in one or two key pieces that embody that style while maintaining your classic and chic basics.

If you build your wardrobe with a series of classic pieces such as the well-fitting tailored dark bottoms, crispy white shirt, and the like, you can use these pieces as the canvas on which to decorate and accent with the new and trendy pieces.

If you buy these pieces in timeless styles then they will move with you through future fashion trends. If however, you build your entire wardrobe every season with the trendiest and most fashionable pieces, you will soon find that your entire wardrobe is dated and looks old.

Keeping classic lines as your staples and adding trendy pieces will keep your wardrobe fresh and up-to-date.

Keep your classic pieces in good repair; dry clean them when necessary; tend to stains and tears immediately to avoid further damage; and hang or fold your clothes properly to prevent creasing and wrinkles.

Update your old clothing by adding in new and interesting accessories. Your same black dress in a classic cut will look stylish and on trend again when you incorporate some hot and chic accessories.

Your old classic cut jeans will instantly look new again when you pair them with a flirty, flow, and floral tunic in this season's muted pastel colors and metallic Grecian inspired sandals.

Take your signature hair style to the next level by adding in feathers or floral hair pins or clips to spotlight this season's trends.

By changing out your old tired sunglasses for this season's fabulous cat's eye frames and a hot neon bag, last year's jacket will be fresh and new again.

How to Stylishly Use Your Old Accessories

Invest your hard-earned money in pieces that you love and will want to use for more than one season. Going uber trendy will date your pieces, but choosing pieces with subtle influences will help you extend their lifespan for more than just one season.

Chapter 9: Conclusion

Your own personal style is one of the most important things that you can develop on your own. To be chic and stylish means that you conform to current style and dress in nice clothing: Stylish is a state of mind.

Invest in and wear flattering basics in your wardrobe. These are pieces that look good on you, but more importantly, make you feel good.

Flattering basics will highlight your best assets and downplay the areas you aren't as proud of.

Know what looks good on you and embrace those styles. Skinny jeans are very hot right now, but someone who is very wide in the hips may not be comfortable wearing these. If you are not comfortable in the clothing you are wearing that will translate into visibly lowered self-confidence.

Get a second opinion about what works on your body type and what does not. Ask your friends, your family, store associates and anyone you may trust. Be prepared for their answers. If you are in tune with what works for you then you probably won't be surprised by their answers, but if you have been living in denial about your size, age and body shape then you may not like what you are going to hear.

Wear sensible and stylish shoes. Keeping your feet happy is the number one way to make it through the day with a smile on your face! Happy and comfortable feet will help carry you through from your morning commute to after dinner drinks and dancing with friends. Unhappy feet will quickly sour your mood and no matter how fashionably and stylishly you are dressed, an angry face will ruin the image.

Find fitted jackets and coats. Many women do not like to wear jackets and coats that are fitted because they believe that they make them look bigger than they are. The truth is just the opposite. Wearing big bulky, cumbersome jackets and coats will add pounds to your silhouette, while a tailored fitted jacket can streamline your shape.

Cardigans are a fantastic way to update your style and help you transition your styles from spring and summer into fall and winter. A fashionable cardigan can take your summer cardigan into winter in a lovely layering piece.

Keep your accessories to a minimum. There are tons of fantastic accessories out there that you are bound to fall in love with. Make sure to only highlight one of them at a time. Key statement pieces are excellent investments and make a fashionable addition to your wardrobe, but by wearing more than one at a time they no longer pop on your outfit, they begin to compete with each other for attention.

Wear the bold cuff bracelet with your black ensemble today and then again with the fashionable scarf you love another day to create two distinctly different outfits.

Use your makeup as an accessory accordingly. If you are using key statement pieces on your wardrobe, then keep your makeup light. Having too many statement pieces (including makeup and accessories) will have your outfit competing against itself and will take away from the chic and stylish lines you are creating.

Wear a fashion forward attitude. Think about the models you see on the runway or in magazines. The outfits they are modelling do not always look fantastic on them. In fact, sometimes those outfits are no more than a burlap bag with a fashionable belt. The difference is that when those models strut their stuff on the runway, they feel beautiful and empowered.

If you do not love yourself, then no amount of fashionable clothing, chic and stylish accessories or fun and fashionable hair styles will mask that. Take some time to focus on yourself and remember what you love about the way you look. Maybe it's your smile or the shapeliness of your legs. Perhaps you love the way your waist cinches in just so at your hip or the way your eyes sparkle when you're excited. Find that part of you that you love and spend time with it. You will soon find that you have many other fine attributes that deserve your love!

Fashion is a very personal expression. It is one way that you can let the world see who you are deep down inside. Your own personal style can and should be subtly guided and influenced by what is hot and happening in the fashion world today. Resist the temptation to bathe in the current fashions, though, because you will quickly lose your own personal style and look like a cookie cutter fashion plate with no individual representation of your own.

Be true to yourself when you are thinking about fashion, but be open to taking some daring and unique fashion risks. If you follow the trends to the letter then you will end up looking just like everyone else in the fashion world, and you will lose your individual style.

Open your stylized life up to some variety. If you are a traditional pant wearer, then spend some time looking at other options. If you are a streamlined dresser who prefers the clean cut lines of jackets and pants then consider a ruffled piece that might soften your style and add a new dimension that you may just love.

If you notice a color trend in your closet (for example, your clothes are all represented in a sea of neutral beige, browns, blues and blacks), open your mind to trying a pop of color in your wardrobe with a bubble gum pint tunic or color blocked sheath dress.

You should have more than one pair of denims in your repertoire. A dressy pair will take you out for dinner and to other social engagements while a casual pair will get you through the weekend and a very relaxed pair will carry you through your outdoor events. Remember to try them on because every cut, style, and brand fits differently.

Everyone will fall victims to impulse buy at some point in their lives. But if you plan out your wardrobe and always have an understanding of what you have in your closet and how things will work together, you can sometimes avoid the temptation. Always think to yourself how many other items you have at home that you can wear this piece with. If the answer is less than two and you are not otherwise in love with it, it might not be a good investment.

Knowing what you have on hand can also help you plan on the best ways to mix and match your current wardrobe with seasonal pieces that will keep you looking stylish and chic from one season to the next.

Sometimes when you are shopping it is better to go for quality over quantity. If you invest money in a classic quality piece that will last you for many seasons then it could end up being a better deal for you than buying the same item four times over because it is of inferior quality and keeps falling apart, or because it is super trendy and becomes outdated before the season is over.

If you are on a fashion budget, then be sure to check out all of the unorthodox fashion places you and your friends know of. Consignment stores offer gently used brand name fashions at a greatly reduced price. In addition, you can sell some of the items you don't love anymore there and get some money back to update your wardrobe with some new "must have" pieces.

Thrift stores such as the Salvation Army may become more of a treasure hunt for you because they are not as selective about the clothing they take in, but oftentimes with a little patience and perseverance, you can find some really fashionable treasures that would be a fantastic addition to your current wardrobe.

Style shouldn't be expensive, so keep your eyes peeled for sales, discounts and other cost savings promotions.

When you are looking at nail polish colors and designs do not fall into the matchy-matchy trap. Your nail polish is meant to compliment your outfit selection and not match it exactly. Your nails are another great way to add an interesting and stylish punch of color or unexpected designs.

Give yourself a final look when you are dressed and evaluate the final product. A stylish and chic woman does not show too much skin. A little skin is sexy and fun. A lot of skin can quickly become trashy and cheap.

If you choose to show some skin in the cleavage area, back, arms, legs, or midriff keeps it looking classy and sophisticated to prevent you from looking like one of the cast members of Jersey shores. While these women are unmistakably beautiful and often on trend, their interpretation of the day's styles often end up with them exposing too much skin which detracts from their stylish fashions and takes them from what could have been a very stylish ensemble and makes it tacky.

Don't try too hard. Fashion and style should be effortless, or at least look like it is. If you're trying too hard to incorporate the latest trends and styles then you quickly move from being a strong fashion forward female to a little girl playing dress up in her mother's clothing where nothing fits just right and it all seems like it is too much.

Make sure that the entire package goes together. If you are wearing an outfit that is dressy and stylish, then make sure that your hair reflects the same image.

Ponytails are quick and easy to do and with the right accessories they can become quite fashionable and stylish. Messy and unclean hair will always look untidy, so be sure that no matter what you do with your hair it is clean and tidy.

No matter what styles you choose to reflect your stylish and chic image, remember that that most important style accessory you can wear is your confidence. Be brave. Be bold. Be beautiful. Be you!